# COMPETITION AND COMPASSION

## Conflicting Roles for Public Hospitals

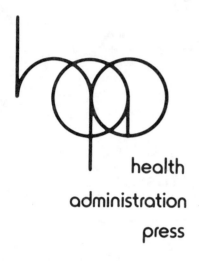

health
administration
press

# COMPETITION AND COMPASSION

## Conflicting Roles for Public Hospitals

Stuart H. Altman, Charles Brecher,
Mary G. Henderson, and
Kenneth E. Thorpe, Editors

Health Administration Press
Ann Arbor, Michigan 1989

**Library of Congress Cataloging-in-Publication Data**

Competition and compassion.

   Includes index.
   1. Hospitals, Public — United States — Administration.  2. Hospitals, Public — United States — Finance.  I. Altman, Stuart H. [DNLM: 1. Governing Board — organization & administration — United States. 2. Hospitals, Public — organization & administration — United States. 3. Hospitals, Teaching — United States.   4. Marketing of Health Services — United States. WX 27 AA1 C73]
   RA971.C72   1989   362.1'1'068      88-32066
   ISBN 0-910701-37-7


Health Administration Press
A Division of the Foundation of the
   American College of Healthcare Executives
1021 East Huron Street
Ann Arbor, Michigan 48104-9990
(313)764-1380

# Table of Contents

# List of Tables

# Preface

This book was inspired by Dr. James G. Hirsch, the late president of the Josiah Macy, Jr. Foundation. Throughout his distinguished career, Dr. Hirsch was concerned with the capacity of the American health care system to meet the needs of the urban poor. After assuming leadership of the Foundation, he focused on the municipal hospitals of New York City. In the early 1980s Dr. Hirsch began to raise a series of questions about the effectiveness of policies developed in the 1960s for the management of municipal hospitals. To stimulate consideration of the problem in its broadest context, he and his associate, Maxine Bleich, began discussions in the academic community about ways to assess public hospital performance and to identify approaches that might lead to improved performance.

One consequence of Dr. Hirsch's concern was a research proposal prepared jointly by the Heller School of Brandeis University and the Citizens Budget Commission in New York City. We felt the issue was relevant in communities other than New York and that objective analysis of public hospital performance ought to be framed in a conceptual approach with national applicability. Our approach, supported by a grant from the Josiah Macy, Jr. Foundation in early 1985, was to examine policies relating to the governance, finance, and medical staffing of public hospitals through a series of case studies spanning the period 1980–84. The assumption was that by evaluating the effects of changes implemented just before or during this period we could learn much about how different governance structures, financing practices, and affiliation arrangements altered hospital performance.

Early in the study period we became aware of a data base relating to all hospitals in the nation's largest cities and were able, through the cooperation of the American Hospital Association and Judith Feder and Jack Hadley of the Urban Institute (and now both at Georgetown

University), to use that data base to explore these issues with greater statistical rigor. We believe the combined approach proved fruitful, and the contents of this book are the evidence. For stimulating our interest and providing financial as well as intellectual support we thank the Board of the Josiah Macy, Jr. Foundation and Maxine Bleich, and gratefully acknowledge the help of the late James Hirsch.

To implement the study required the cooperation and talent of many people. While Raymond D. Horton, President of the Citizens Budget Commission, does not appear as a coauthor or coeditor of this volume, he served in many ways to make the book a reality. He assisted in the planning of the study as well as its implementation and kept raising fundamental questions that enhanced the chapter authors' abilities to make insightful observations.

Both the Heller School and the Citizens Budget Commission were fortunate in finding able researchers to collaborate on the study. At the Heller School initial work was done by Sally Bachman and Dennis Beatrice, but newly emerging responsibilities required their energies. They were replaced by Mary Henderson, who coordinated the efforts in Massachusetts, and two able researchers, Martha Solish and Joel Weissman. The latter assumed responsibility for preparing the case studies in Los Angeles and Tampa. Mary not only completed the case study in Memphis, she also played a key role in refining the initial conceptual framework presented in Chapter 2 and in drafting the Introduction. At the Citizens Budget Commission, we were fortunate in having the help of Cynthia Green, a research associate, in preparing the New York City case study, and in recruiting Kenneth Thorpe, then of Columbia University and now at Harvard, to undertake a comparative statistical analysis and help in the local research. The substantial contributions of Kenneth Thorpe and Mary Henderson in shaping the analysis and putting in the extra effort to produce this book are reflected in their due credit as coeditors of the volume as well as coauthors of particular chapters.

Completing the case studies also required the cooperation of the leadership of the institutions studied. In Los Angeles, Memphis, and Tampa, this cooperation was graciously provided and we were able to conduct structured interviews with key individuals as well as obtain unpublished financial reports and other data. In addition, representatives from each of these hospitals reviewed drafts of the case studies and provided many helpful suggestions. We are sincerely grateful for this cooperation, although the authors and editors are responsible for any remaining errors or misinterpretations.

In New York the city's top political leadership was less receptive to an outside examination of the Health and Hospitals Corporation.

However, once the book was drafted, we shared a copy with Dr. Jo Ivey Boufford, President of the Health and Hospitals Corporation. She and her staff then provided many helpful suggestions (although, again, the authors and editors are responsible for any remaining errors in fact or interpretation).

Many other groups concerned with public hospitals also provided advice. Dr. Dennis Andrulis, Vice President of the National Association of Public Hospitals, was especially generous with his time and made available the resources of his organization.

The marked-up versions of the individual chapters were converted into a coherent and legible manuscript thanks to the efforts of Mary De La Fuente and Fondia Thompson, the secretarial staff of the Citizens Budget Commission. They put all the typescript into a common word processing package and updated these master copies through the waves of revisions. This process was ably overseen by Barbara Weinstein, the Commission's Vice President for Administration.

Once the complete book was ready, we submitted it to the Health Administration Press. Their anonymous reviewers prepared detailed and helpful comments to which all of the authors were good enough to take the time to respond even though they had moved on to new assignments. The result was a much improved version. Similarly, the careful copyediting by the Health Administration Press helped eliminate many errors or potential sources of confusion. Once all the queries and comments were accounted for, the staff of the Health Administration Press expedited the production of the book. While the entire process of review, revision, and production took longer than the editors and sponsors initially anticipated, we are confident the result is an important book.

Stuart H. Altman
Charles Brecher
September 26, 1988

# ఆ 1 ి

# *Introduction*

## Stuart H. Altman and Mary G. Henderson

Debate over the future of urban public hospitals is not new. In the early 1970s, considerable attention focused on the problems of these institutions. Numerous studies, task force reports, and magazine articles depicted urban public hospitals as financially stressed, obsolete deliverers of second-class health care to the poor. But in spite of the wide range of strategies that were proposed to address these shortcomings, most of the underlying problems remain a decade later, exacerbated by national economic conditions and by shifts in federal policy that have reduced support for health care and social programs. Meanwhile, ironically, the same economic and political forces that undermine the viability of urban public hospitals contribute to increased demand for their services.

Although they serve Americans at all income levels, the fundamental mission of urban public hospitals is to care for the uninsured and indigent. An estimated 23 million Americans have no public or private insurance coverage, and millions more do not have coverage during some portion of each year.[1] The uninsured include, in addition to those who have low incomes yet are not eligible for Medicaid, patients with catastrophic illnesses who exhaust their insurance benefits, many self-employed individuals, employees of small businesses that do not provide health insurance, and people unable because of preexisting medical conditions to obtain insurance.

Public hospitals provide most of the care for these uninsured patients. A 1980 survey found that nonfederal public hospitals, which make up about one-third of the nation's community hospitals, accounted for 43 percent of all bad debt and charity care.[2] In place of national health insurance, the nation has substituted a network of public hospitals as a less costly surrogate. This network constitutes an implicit acknowledgment that, due to economic circumstances or special health needs, a significant proportion of the population falls between the cracks of the current health insurance system.

Urban public hospitals also provide many services not offered by private institutions. They provide disproportionately large shares of primary care, often in conjunction with community-based health centers. Care for social-medical problems, such as alcoholism and drug abuse, is also typically provided by these institutions. In many cases, urban public hospitals have developed into large-scale institutions, not because of a need for sophisticated, technologically advanced services, but rather because of the intense need for basic services in large cities.[3]

The first section of this chapter describes more fully the role of urban public hospitals as caregivers. The next two sections review the long-standing problems of urban public hospitals, discuss more recent developments including increasingly hostile federal policy and a more competitive private health care industry, and describe some new initiatives that have the potential to improve the status of public hospitals. The fourth section of this chapter outlines some options available to urban public hospitals in responding to their problems. These choices relate to how public hospitals govern themselves, how they structure their teaching affiliations, and whether or not they compete for insured patients. The remainder of the book, outlined in the final section of this chapter, provides evidence for the advantages and disadvantages of each strategy.

## The Importance of Urban Public Hospitals

Urban public hospitals, the subject of so much debate and concern, are only a small minority of the approximately 1,700 nonfederal public hospitals in the United States. In 1978 the Commission on Public General Hospitals reported that only 90 hospitals, or just under 5 percent of all local public hospitals, were located in large cities. These 90 hospitals were concentrated in 63 of the nation's 100 largest cities.[4] By 1985, because of closures and transfers of ownership, only about 60 of these hospitals, located in 48 of the 100 largest cities, remained. These institutions are large, averaging about 500 beds; they also are major teaching institutions.[5]

The commission characterized these urban public hospitals as serving patients who have no other source of health care and "as a group [having] the most serious and persistent problems."[6] Their two major groups of patients are Medicaid enrollees and uninsured indigents. Approximately 25 percent of the total revenues of these hospitals is from Medicaid; 30 percent is from state and local government appropriations earmarked to support indigent care.[7] While private institutions provide the greater proportion (70 percent) of Medicaid-financed care, charity care is overwhelmingly the responsibility of the urban public hospitals, which provide fully 65 percent of all charity care in the nation's 100 largest cities.[8]

Urban public hospitals are significant providers of ambulatory services. The Commission on Public General Hospitals found that public hospitals in the nation's 100 largest cities provided 45 percent of all hospital-based ambulatory care visits, including 28 percent of all emergency room visits. Urban public hospitals also provide disproportionately large volumes of other services. The commission found that these hospitals accounted for 42 percent of all burn units, one-fourth of all hospital-based alcoholism treatment programs, one-fourth of all neonatal intensive care units, and one-fifth of all psychiatric emergency and psychiatric inpatient care units. Urban public hospitals are frequently the site of care for victims of crime and life-threatening trauma. Because of the hospitals' ties to local government, they generally are able to coordinate these services with related public functions, such as fire, police, and ambulance services.[9]

Finally, urban public hospitals are responsible for training a significant proportion of the country's health care professionals. These institutions represent less than 5 percent of total hospital beds, but they train about one-fifth of all medical and dental residents and one-tenth of other health professionals.[10] Because some of their services are specialized, urban public hospitals often provide important training opportunities in many kinds of care. Because of their unique case load and service mix, urban public hospitals face a more uncertain future than either other public hospitals or private institutions.

## A Historical Perspective

Most of the problems besetting urban public hospitals are rooted in the origins of these hospitals as institutions responsible for the poor. Many modern urban public hospitals are descendants of late eighteenth-century workhouses or almshouses. Under the jurisdiction of local governments, almshouses began to offer rudimentary medical care to residents and, in some cases, to poor people from outside the almshouse. In the late eighteenth and early nineteenth centuries, the infirmaries became independent from the almshouses but remained supported by local tax dollars. Conditions in these infirmaries were usually abominable: individuals with acute and chronic medical and psychological problems were mixed together, looked after by caretakers with little training or equipment.

The reform movement of the mid-1800s provided the impetus for local governments to become more heavily involved in providing medical care to the poor. States began to subsidize local governments in the establishment of public general hospitals. By 1943, about 655 of these hospitals had been established nationwide, containing almost 10 percent of all the beds in the country and accounting for almost 11 percent of all admissions. The financing of these hospitals was not helped greatly by the federal government, however, until the enactment of Medicare and Medicaid in 1965. Under the Social Security Act of 1935, states were not able to use federal funds to pay local public hospitals for care; all welfare benefits had to be paid in cash directly to the recipient, not provided as in-kind services.

Although local public hospitals became the most widely used place of care for the poor between 1930 and 1950, private institutions also became increasingly involved in caring for the indigent. This was especially true in New York and some other large cities where local government paid substantial amounts to private hospitals for indigent care. Nevertheless, local public hospitals thrived in this period with support from public health advocates, philanthropists, and public administrators. Federal financial aid for construction and renovation came from the Public Works Administration and the Works Progress Administration.

During this period the prestige of many urban public hospitals was enhanced by links to medical schools, which saw in the urban public hospitals reservoirs of research and teaching "material." Many of the teaching physicians had reputations as excellent researchers; their presence enhanced the reputation of the hospitals, which led to increased support from local officials and the public.

After 1950, the vitality of many urban public hospitals began to decline sharply. Four major factors worked synergistically to cause this.[11] First, the population served by the hospitals became increasingly poor and dependent. With the advent and rapid spread of private health insurance through employment after World War II, middle-class and unionized workers could, and did, begin to choose private hospitals over public ones. The middle class also began to migrate in large numbers to the suburbs, leaving the inner cities to the poor. This phenomenon led to the second major factor, the fiscal deterioration of city governments.

Because the departure of the middle class (and its replacement by service-needy populations) eroded their tax bases, local governments could no longer afford to support public hospitals at previous levels. The problem was compounded by rapid cost increases in hospital care, which created great budgetary pressures. Although the passage of Medicare and Medicaid in 1965 undoubtedly helped the public hospitals, many of the poor have never been covered by these programs. Currently the share of the poor covered by Medicaid is only about 34 percent.[12]

Third, urban public hospitals lost leading medical research staff and faculty during the 1950s, a period when many new, generous research grants went primarily to prestigious, privately endowed medical schools and teaching hospitals and to state university medical schools and teaching hospitals. Urban public hospitals then had difficulty attracting medical staff, and the quality of staff and facilities deteriorated so sharply that many of the hospitals were in danger of losing accreditation.

Finally, the demand for hospital services changed. After World War II, the urban poor's expectations about the accessibility and quality of primary care had risen. When many office-based physicians followed the middle class to the suburbs, the burden of providing much of this ambulatory care fell on the urban public hospitals, at a time when these hospitals' resources were constrained. Exacerbating this problem was the tendency for public and private insurance programs to pay less favorably for outpatient services than for inpatient care. Moreover, public hospitals experienced declines in inpatient occupancy rate after the enactment of Medicare and Medicaid, because these programs gave some poor people the opportunity to obtain private hospital care.

Some observers in the 1970s attributed the problems of urban public hospitals to control by local government. These observers believed that antiquated civil service procedures and the sometimes complicated purchasing requirements imposed by governing bodies were impeding the efficiency of hospital management. They also claimed that the potential for political intervention in the day-to-day affairs of the hospital decreased the professional autonomy of hospital administrators.

Local government hospitals were also believed to be at a disadvantage relative to private hospitals in their access to capital funds. Although public hospitals appear to have an advantage because of the favorable borrowing power of state and local governments, many of these governing bodies reached their legal borrowing limits in the 1970s. Even where the limit had not been reached, urban public hospitals were still obliged to compete with many projects unrelated to health for approval of proposed bond issues. Moreover, private hospitals have actually enjoyed government subsidies (not requiring local voter approval) for capital expenditures because they often may borrow through tax-exempt revenue bonds.

## The Current Situation

In the 1980s many of the long-standing problems of urban public hospitals have worsened and new ones have surfaced. Several states and the business communities in some areas have recognized, however, that the public hospital can be an essential component of the health care system. Business communities and states are beginning to play a significant role in reshaping service delivery arrangements and developing solutions to many of the problems faced by urban public hospitals.

The undercapitalization of public hospitals remains a significant difficulty. Cutbacks in Medicaid eligibility, coupled with severe unemployment and an influx of undocumented aliens, have led to growing numbers of uninsured urban residents. Reports of the transfer or "dumping" of these uninsured patients from private to public hospitals have become frequent.[13]

While private hospitals are shifting more of the costs of treating the poor to local governments, urban public hospitals are finding it increasingly difficult to cover costs by "cost shifting" to Medicare or private insurance. Payments under Medicare's diagnosis-related group (DRG) system are alleged to be inadequate, in many cases, for the types of patient frequently seen in urban public hospitals. With growing competition among private insurers for the corporate health care dollar, urban public hospitals, which are high-cost providers, are at a disadvantage in participating in alternative delivery systems such as preferred provider organizations (PPOs) and health maintenance organizations (HMOs).

### Growing Numbers of the Uninsured

One of the major initiatives of the Reagan administration was the Omnibus Reconciliation Act of 1981, which included phased-in cutbacks in federal Medicaid payments to states. These reductions, reaching 4.5 percent in fiscal year 1984, significantly worsened the budgetary problems states were already experiencing with their Medicaid programs. The dual consequences were benefit limitations and tightening of eligibility requirements, both of which have had particularly harmful effects on urban public hospitals. Increased eligibility restrictions have disqualified many people who formerly qualified for Medicaid. These uninsured are significantly more likely to do without needed care than those with insurance, thus increasing the probability that they will be sicker when they finally obtain care.[14]

And when the uninsured do seek care it is likely to be at a public institution. Public hospitals devoted almost 40 percent of their resources to care for the poor in 1980 while private hospitals devoted only 12 percent of their resources to such care.[15] The necessary reliance of the uninsured on public hospitals is highlighted in a 1983 survey that found that 44 percent of the newly unemployed (and uninsured) patients of public hospitals had not used these hospitals as a regular source of care before becoming unemployed.[16]

Benefit reductions under Medicaid have also adversely affected public hospitals. Limiting the number of reimbursable days of hospital care harshly penalizes public hospitals in particular, because average lengths of stay are longer in public than in private facilities. These limitations also increase the financial incentives for private hospitals to dump Medicaid patients who are unusually sick and require more than the allowable number of days of care. Cutbacks in services covered under Medicaid, such as outpatient, mental health, and drug abuse and alcoholism services, have similar harmful repercussions for the public hospitals, which play a disproportionately large role in providing this care.

On the positive side, some communities have received governmental and philanthropic support to develop alternative delivery systems for the indigent that can lessen the need for substantial new funding. Several public hospitals, including Boston City Hospital, Metropolitan Hospital in New York City, and Jackson Memorial Hospital in Miami, have recently established case management programs for the indigent, in which all care is monitored by a medical team. Although the cost-effectiveness of these case management arrangements has not yet been demonstrated, they are considered to increase the probability that care will be delivered more appropriately and efficiently, thus allowing a greater number of the uninsured to be served.

## Changes in Medicare Policy

Changes in payment for care under the federal Medicare program also affect urban public hospitals negatively. The private sector readily accepted Medicare beneficiaries in the past, but the DRG payment system enacted in 1983 has made it "unprofitable" to treat some of the elderly who have more costly conditions. These patients have become candidates for transfers to public hospitals. As a result, Medicare patients treated in public hospitals may now be sicker than their private hospital counterparts. Specifically, for similar diagnoses, the public hospital patients are more likely to have complications and to be outliers (i.e., to have significantly longer than average lengths of stay). Both these factors contribute to the higher than average costs by diagnosis seen in public hospitals.[17] An analysis of the effect of the DRG payment methodology on 27 public hospitals indicated that in the first year of the system, average Medicare revenues decreased almost $2.5 million, while average Medicare costs increased $1.1 million.[18]

Congress recently passed legislation that lets hospitals that treat large numbers of low-income patients obtain increased Medicare payments under the DRG system. The 1986 Budget Reconciliation Amendment allows hospitals with a disproportionate share of Medicaid patients to receive as much as a 15 percent add-on to their DRG payment levels. This legislation is similar to language in the 1981 Omnibus Reconciliation Act that provided a mechanism to increase Medicaid funding to hospitals with a disproportionate share of low-income patients. Although some states have taken advantage of this Medicaid option, many have been able to avoid increasing Medicaid payment rates to these "disproportionate share" hospitals because the Health Care Financing Administration (HCFA) has allowed states broad discretion in their interpretation of this legislation. Nevertheless, urban public hospitals stand to be major beneficiaries of these Medicaid and Medicare reforms.

Payment for capital costs under Medicaid has become a contentious issue as the federal government grapples with finding an efficient and equitable way to fund the depreciation and debt service expenses of health care facilities. As noted earlier, most public hospitals operate with deteriorating and outmoded physical plants. Their mix of uninsured and publicly funded patients greatly hinders their ability to compete for capital in the bond market. There is an inverse relationship between a hospital's bond rating and the proportion of its revenue derived from Medicaid and Medicare.[19] Urban public hospitals, with roughly 40 percent of their revenues from these sources, suffer a distinct disadvantage. Payments for capital costs accounted for 6 percent of Medicare reimbursements to all hospitals with over 400 beds in 1981 but averaged only 3.9 percent to urban public hospitals of similar size.[20] The lack of resources for capital investments and the need to use a large proportion of their discretionary funds to cover operating deficits caused public hospitals to have a lower rate of increase in capital expenditures (5 percent) than private not-for-profit (16 percent) and proprietary (12 percent) hospitals in the late 1970s.[21] This lack of capital investment is bearing its fruits in the 1980s in the form of inefficient physical plants, outmoded equipment, and a lack of amenities.

The Reagan administration's health policies under Medicare and other programs have sought to increase competition in the industry as a mechanism to control costs. These procompetition policies encourage insurance plans to bargain with hospitals over hospital charges and to seek lower prices for their subscribers.

Critics of this approach point out that the competition proposals jeopardize poor people's access to care by threatening the institutions that provide most of their care — the public hospitals. That public hospitals have higher than average costs is probably due to an indeterminate combination of operating inefficiencies and a sicker, more complex patient mix. Because of these higher costs, public hospitals are less able to compete for inclusion in PPOs, HMOs, or other alternative delivery system models. This causes the public hospitals to lose their private patients and encourages private hospitals not to treat the less economically viable patient.

## *Options for Urban Public Hospitals*

Urban public hospitals confront perhaps the most difficult period in their history. These hospitals and their government sponsors do have several broad options, however — in the absence of major national reforms in the way hospital care is financed — to improve their future performance. These policy options relate to governance structures, financing arrangements, teaching affiliations, and market strategies.

In the late 1960s and early 1970s, several local governments tried integrating the local public health department, the local public hospital, and other local publicly funded services under a single health services agency. A major impetus behind these mergers was a desire to improve local governmental efficiency by consolidating functions under one auspice.[22] A second type of governance change also undertaken to improve efficiency has been to transfer the governance of the hospital from a local government to a new, more politically autonomous structure. The purpose of this change is to free the hospital administration from the constraints imposed by civil service and other bureaucratic norms and to avoid potential political interference in routine hospital operations. The new governance arrangement is often introduced in tandem with new management personnel.

Chapter 2 reviews the available evidence about the effect of both such governance changes. The effect of mergers has been more extensively studied than that of governance transfer to a nonpublic entity.

Although anecdotal accounts are common, little systematic data have been generated on how this latter type of change affects the efficiency of the institutions, the quality of their services, or poor people's access to care. This book addresses the subject through case studies and other analyses.

Teaching affiliations undoubtedly have helped to establish the reputation of many public hospitals as high quality institutions and to ensure that they acquire the medical staff they need. However, there are also disadvantages to teaching affiliations. Increased operating costs appear to be associated with teaching, and there may be a risk that patients used as clinical material will be treated in a dehumanizing way, as "guinea pigs." Furthermore, when a public hospital and a private teaching hospital share medical staff, the staff's allegiance generally is to the "home" teaching hospital to which they make private referrals; this can work to the disadvantage of the public hospital.

At least some urban public hospitals may soon reevaluate their teaching relationships. New arrangements may be sought in which nonacademic, community physicians would play a greater role in patient care and policymaking at public hospitals. Some hospitals may even consider contracting with private physician groups to provide care, instead of using teaching physicians and residents. This book compares urban public hospitals that have different types of teaching affiliation to determine whether and how new relationships might improve public hospital performance.

Although some analysts believe that the only solution to the problems of urban public hospitals is universal health insurance, other financing options are available in the interim. As an alternative to continued reliance on subsidies from local governments, urban public hospitals could compete for the privately insured and shift some uncompensated care costs to private insurers.

Either or both of these options may be feasible for some urban public hospitals, but each presents problems for many hospitals. Public funds are increasingly difficult to obtain. Tax dollars are scarce, and support for care to the uninsured must compete with a myriad of other public services for taxpayer approval. Cost shifting to private insurers is also increasingly difficult. As businesses face intensified pressure to control the health care costs of their employees, they increase the competition among private insurers to lower premiums. The insurers, in turn, seek to reduce the amounts paid to hospitals and thus effectively lower revenues per patient. Thus, even hospitals with a favorable payer mix will find it increasingly difficult to shift their charity care costs. Urban public hospitals will face even greater difficulty, since they already have a relatively small base of privately insured patients.

Several types of payment reform have recently been enacted to improve the financial status of urban public hospitals. In some areas, care for the uninsured is financed through grants from philanthropic groups. In others, the business community has directly supported care for the indigent and has sponsored health insurance initiatives for people who are employed but uninsured and for the newly unemployed. Some states have begun or are considering earmarked taxes to pay for indigent care. Some localities have started pooling arrangements whereby all hospitals or insurers are expected to contribute to the financing of indigent care on some predetermined basis.

Although these financing reforms are fragmented and generally inadequate to address fully the fiscal distress of many of the nation's urban public hospitals, they are widely regarded as steps in the right direction. Hospitals benefiting from these reforms will also continue to rely on local, state, and federal subsidies. Hospitals that cannot or will not seek greater subsidies for indigent care will become players in the ever more competitive market for the privately insured. This book provides evidence by which to assess the effects of relying on one or the other strategy on the performance of urban public hospitals.

Closely related to governance and financing options are changes in a public hospital's market strategy, that is, the position it seeks to attain in the local health care market. The merger option (also known as vertical integration), exemplified by the Denver public hospital system, involves continued reliance on government subsidies. The local government integrates its health care resources — the public hospital, public health clinics, and other publicly funded services — into a single system. Community health centers delivering primary care make up the core of the system, and the hospital is operated as an inpatient and specialty consultation backup facility. Integrated, comprehensive, and accessible patient care is the primary goal of such a system; teaching and research are not high priorities. According to one expert observer, the Denver experience shows that an integrated system can work, but that adequate funding, committed local leadership, and the willingness of professionals to collaborate and cooperate are essential to its success.[23]

Alternatively, urban public hospitals can market themselves to all sectors of the community, including the privately insured. The attractions of this option are that it removes the stigma attached to public institutions as providers of last resort and offers the poor the same standard of care provided to the more wealthy. However, many hospitals' ability to follow this course is severely hampered by the problems already discussed: they are at a competitive disadvantage in attracting private patients and private physicians because they are unable to provide advanced medical technology, plush patient accommodations, and high quality support services. Despite these obstacles, some urban public hospitals have launched aggressive campaigns to market themselves to the insured. This book includes analyses of two public hospital systems—Tampa and Memphis—that opted for the competitive strategy. Their experience is compared with that of two systems that remained more dependent on government subsidies and more committed to serving the indigent—Los Angeles and New York City.

## Plan of the Book

Many studies have documented the plight of urban public hospitals, but few have attempted systematically to identify and assess policies that can help local officials improve the performance of their public hospitals. This book presents the results of such an effort.

Chapter 2 defines the three criteria for assessing the performance of public hospitals: efficiency, quality, and access. In addition, policy options related to the governance structure of the hospital, the nature of its teaching commitment, its financing arrangements, and its market position are identified. Chapter 2 also reviews the available evidence linking the performance criteria and policy options. Finally, this chapter describes the methodology of the study, which consists of case studies of the urban public hospital systems located in New York City, Los Angeles, Tampa, and Memphis and a cross-sectional analysis of hospital systems in the nation's 100 largest cities.

Chapters 3 through 6 present the evidence from these empirical investigations; each chapter presents one of the four case studies, in the order indicated above. Chapter 7 discusses the findings from the cross-sectional analysis. The final chapter synthesizes the results of these complementary approaches to identify some general principles for improving the performance of urban public hospitals.

## Notes

1. E. Richard Brown, "Public Hospitals on the Brink: Their Problems and Their Options," *Journal of Health Politics, Policy and Law* 7 (Winter 1983): 927–44.
2. Jack Hadley and Judith Feder, *Hospitals' Financial Status and Care to the Poor in 1980* (Washington, DC: Urban Institute, 1983).
3. Mary Grogan Brown, "Public-General Hospitals: Important Factors in the Delivery of Patient Care," in Commission on Public-General Hospitals, ed., *Readings on Public General Hospitals* (Chicago: Hospital Research and Educational Trust, 1978), pp. 1–88.

4. Ibid.
5. Ibid.
6. Ibid., p. 8.
7. Dennis P. Andrulis, "Survival Strategies for Public Hospitals," *Business and Health* 3, no. 7 (June 1986): 31–36.
8. Hadley and Feder, *Hospitals' Financial Status*.
9. Brown, "Public-General Hospitals."
10. Ibid.
11. William Shonick, "Early Developments and Recent Trends in the Evolution of the Local Public Hospital," *American Review of Public Health* 5 (1984): 53–81.
12. Health Care Financing Administration, *Health Care Financing Program Statistics* (Baltimore: U.S. Department of Health and Human Services, August 1985), p. 152.
13. Robert Sillen, Statement to the Subcommittee on Health, Committee on Finance, United States Senate, Washington, DC, 9 March 1984.
14. Ibid.
15. Hadley and Feder, *Hospitals' Financial Status*.
16. Results from 1983 National Association of Public Hospitals Survey, cited in Sillen, Statement to the Subcommittee on Health.
17. Michael Schwartz, Jeffrey Merrill, and G. B. Klebanoff, "DRG Based Case Mix and Public Hospitals," *Medical Care* 22 (1984): 283–99.
18. Results from 1983 National Association of Public Hospitals Survey, cited in Sillen, Statement to the Subcommittee on Health.
19. Sillen, Statement to the Subcommittee on Health.
20. Gerard Anderson and Paul B. Ginsburg, "Prospective Capital Payments to Hospitals," *Health Affairs* 2, no. 3 (Fall 1983): 52–63.
21. Eleanor Kinney and Bonnie Lefkowitz, "Capital Cost Reimbursement to Community Hospitals Under Federal Health Insurance Programs," *Journal of Health Politics, Policy and Law* 7, no. 3 (Fall 1982): 648–66.
22. William Shonick, "Mergers of Public Health Departments with Public Hospitals in Urban Areas: Findings of 12 Field Studies," *Medical Care*, supplement (August 1980): 1–50.
23. Ibid.

# ⁓ 2 ⁓

# Conceptual Model and Methods

Mary G. Henderson, Kenneth E. Thorpe, and Charles Brecher

The basic purpose of this study is to uncover the underlying relationships between hospital performance and the policies available to local officials who manage public hospitals. This task requires an objective set of criteria for assessing hospital performance, the identification of specific policy options, and the presentation of evidence that links the policy options to the performance criteria.

This chapter presents the performance criteria and policy options that are analyzed and specifies the types of evidence to be considered in assessing the effectiveness of the options. The first section identifies three performance criteria—efficiency, quality, and access. These criteria are then related to policy decisions regarding four aspects of public hospital structure and operations—form of governance, financing arrangements, linkages to teaching institutions, and the market strategy adopted by managers. In addition to indicating the measures used for each criterion, this section draws upon earlier research to elaborate the expected relationships between the policy options and the performance standards.

The second section describes the methods used to assess the actual relationships between policy and performance. Two approaches are outlined—a cross-sectional analysis of hospital systems in the nation's 100 largest cities and detailed case studies of 4 large cities with public hospitals, with emphasis on changes during the 1980–84 period. The characteristics of these 4 cities and their health care institutions are described and the basis for their selection is presented.

## Conceptual Model

Conceptual models relate variables over which some control is exercised (so-called independent variables) to outcomes in which the analyst is interested because of their social importance. Thus, a useful model involves both a set of outcomes or dependent variables and a set of independent variables that are logically and theoretically linked to the dependent variables.

### Dependent Variables

The trinity of efficiency, quality, and access is well established as the set of criteria for assessing health care. However, the specific measures available to gauge these aspects of care are more problematic.

For individual institutions, including public hospitals, efficiency is usually reflected in unit costs. Public hospitals will be judged on the basis of expenses per discharge or expenses per day of care. However, two other important factors must be considered. First, episodes (days or discharges) of hospital care vary in the level of resources required, depending on the condition of the patient. Therefore, before judgments about relative efficiency are made, consideration must be given to variations in case mix and other characteristics of the patients treated. Second, unit costs may vary because of differences in local labor market characteristics that generate different compensation levels for the same quantity and quality of labor. Personnel costs typically represent about two-thirds of all hospital operating costs, so wage differentials can significantly affect relative unit costs. Accordingly, efficiency will also be assessed by focusing on the amount of labor used to produce services. Such measures include the number of full-time-equivalent personnel per day of care or per discharge. It is important to recognize, however, that the sociocultural characteristics of patients treated at public hospitals may cause these patients to require more labor-intensive resources, for example, social workers and interpreters.

Quality of care can be assessed in three different ways: inputs, process, and outcomes. A widely used standard for judging the inputs or resources available to provide care is the periodic review conducted by the Joint Commission on Accreditation of Healthcare Organizations (JCAHO — formerly the Joint Commission on Accreditation of Hospitals).[1] Health care professionals from several disciplines determine whether a hospital's physical plant, staff patterns, and organizational procedures meet the standards set by the American Medical Association, the American Hospital Association, and other groups. Based on these reviews, the hospital is either accredited or denied accreditation because of specific deficiencies. These JCAHO reviews are the principal basis for assessing quality in this study.

Because JCAHO accreditation represents only conformance with minimally accepted standards and relates primarily to input standards, it is useful to consider additional measures of quality relating to process and outcomes. There is general agreement that health outcomes are the most desirable measure of quality; how well a patient does is the ultimate test of quality. However, it also is widely recognized that it is extremely difficult to determine the direct relationship between a medical service and a patient's health. Therefore, output measures generally cannot be relied upon for judgments of quality for public hospitals.

Process measures indicate the extent to which care adheres to norms, such as the administration of effective tests or procedures and conformance with established length of stay. There are no systematic comparative data for these measures, but such indicators were available and are presented for the public hospitals in the selected case studies. The case studies also report on local perceptions of the adequacy of the physical plant and the quality of the treatment process from the patients' perspective when these impressions were documented in newspaper articles or other sources.

Access to care refers to the ease with which patients receive services. Access can be a problem where services are remotely located, but in most large urban centers the principal limitation on access is an inability to pay. Therefore, the most relevant access measures are those indicating ease of access among poor residents of a city. Such access can be considered from both a communitywide and an institution-specific perspective. In the cross-sectional analysis of large cities, access is measured for the community as a whole in terms of utilization rates for the indigent population. In the case studies, access is considered from the perspective of the public hospital and is gauged by the volume of care the hospital provides to Medicaid and uninsured patients.

## Independent or Policy Variables

The efficiency, quality, and access of public hospitals can be affected by four types of policy decisions—those pertaining to their governance, relationship to teaching institutions, finance, and market strategy.

**Governance Structure.** Traditionally, urban public hospitals were owned and operated by local government entities. For a variety of reasons, however, many localities have sought to give their public

## Table 2.1

## Governance of Urban Public Hospital Systems, 1985

| Type of Governance | Number | Percentage |
|---|---|---|
| Unit of local government | | |
|   City hospital | 8 | 19 |
|   County hospital | 19 | 44 |
|   City/county hospital | 2 | 5 |
|   Total local government | 29 | 67 |
| Independent or semi-independent entity | | |
|   Authority or public benefit corporation | 6 | 14 |
|   Hospital district | 6 | 14 |
|   Other independent entity | 2 | 5 |
|   Total independent entity | 14 | 33 |
|   Grand total | 43 | 100 |

Source: Authors' survey of public hospitals in 100 largest cities.

hospitals more autonomy in their operations than conventional governmental agencies would give them. We conducted a combination mail-and-telephone survey in 1985 to determine the nature of the governance arrangements for urban public hospitals.

Among the 100 largest cities in the United States, 47 had local public hospitals, another 21 had state-run institutions, and 29 had no public hospital facilities. Of the 47 cities with local public hospitals, 43 responded to the survey. (Des Moines, Omaha, Indianapolis, and San Francisco did not.) Among the 43 responding cities, the public hospital system consisted of only one facility in 39 cities; the remaining 4 cities had multiple-hospital public systems (New York, Los Angeles, Atlanta, and Tampa). The cities were thus the locations for 56 different hospitals, but these hospitals represented only 43 different governing structures.

Direct governance by a unit of local government was the most common form, existing in 29 of the 43 hospital systems (see Table 2.1). The systems differed with respect to the unit of local government overseeing them. Nineteen, or fully 44 percent, of the systems were owned and directly operated by their counties. City governments owned and directly operated eight, or 19 percent, of the systems. Two public hospital systems, Denver and Nashville, were operated under the joint jurisdiction of city and county.

Each of the remaining 14 public hospital systems was operated by an independent or semi-independent governing structure. Six of these systems, including those in New York and Atlanta, were governed by authorities or public benefit corporations. In each of another 6 cities, a hospital district was established to govern the hospital. Finally, independent entities established by state statute were the governing structures for the remaining 2 cities.

For each of the hospitals with an independent or semi-independent governance structure, the governing entity was a board. For all but one hospital—Northside Hospital in Atlanta—the board members were appointed officials. The appointments were made by the highest elected city or county official except in Jersey City, where the appointments were made by the governor. Northside Hospital's governing board was elected by city residents.

This shift to a form of governance that is partly or fully separated from local general government, and hence more autonomous, is usually intended to improve performance. The theoretical connections between a more autonomous form of governance and each of the three performance criteria can be derived from earlier research and observations of hospital behavior.

*Governance and efficiency.* The relationship between efficiency and governance is widely disputed. Most hypothesized relationships between hospital governance and performance are derived from theories assigning significance to differences in property rights arrangements.[2] These theories are worth considering as a broad framework, but they do not address the specific issue of the relative efficiency of more or less autonomous governance structures within the public sector.

Property rights are rights to the value of future profits resulting from the operation of a hospital. One would expect systematic differences in hospital behavior depending on the degree to which administrators or physicians of hospitals have well-defined stakes in future profits. The extent to which future profits are transferable to hospital administrators or physicians differs by the type of hospital governance. For instance, in proprietary hospitals, owners, administrators, and shareholders all hold well-defined rights to future profits. As a result, these "claimants" have an incentive to establish rules and regulations within the hospital that will maximize the flow of profits. Thus, proprietary hospitals have incentives to produce medical services of a given quality at minimum cost.

The extent to which property rights are well defined in nonprofit hospitals is more questionable. Some would say that administrators, because of their hospitals' nonprofit status, do not have exclusive claim to future profits.[3] Moreover, goals other than profit maximization and cost minimization often motivate the operating decisions of trustees and administrators. In contrast, Pauly and Redisch note that physicians may lay claim to future profits in "nonprofit" hospitals and therefore have incentives to maximize their incomes jointly.[4] Given these incentives, there may be little observed difference in behavior between profit and nonprofit hospitals.

However, property rights theory clearly suggests that public hospitals will be the least efficient. First, there are usually no claimants to future profits — not even physicians. Indeed, physicians with admitting privileges in public hospitals are often salaried and — because of strong teaching affiliations — often view the public institution as their "second home." Second, the organizational mission of most public hospitals is not to maximize the capitalized value of future income. Instead, other missions — such as being the provider of last resort — dictate their actions. Finally, patronage and other political concerns may lead public hospitals (especially those governed as a unit of local government) to place greater value on higher staffing levels than do other hospitals. All three of these factors could lead to higher unit costs than are observed in other hospitals.

Other theories of public sector decision making are consistent with the property rights thesis. A model of bureaucratic behavior advanced by Niskanen indicates that the goal of bureaucratic decision makers is to maximize the agency's budget.[5] Budget maximization rather than cost minimization as an objective function of decision makers suggests that output and cost expansion are methods of adjusting to revenue increases for public agencies. Wolf has postulated a similar budget expansion and cost-increasing behavior among public sector agencies.[6]

Yet differences in unit costs occur among public hospitals. The literature summarized above suggests that the type of governance structure and the associated autonomy from local government could affect hospital behavior and costs. Removing a public hospital from direct government control by establishing a semi-independent board may circumvent rigidities inherent within a bureaucracy and increase hospital efficiency.

While these theories appear convincing, previous empirical investigations of hospital costs do not provide uniform support for the notion that government-run institutions are always less efficient. Becker and Sloan's recent research shows no statistically significant differences in the efficiency and profitability of for-profit, nonprofit, and public hospitals when other factors are controlled.[7] Wolfe and Sherer's more limited study produced similar results that appear to refute the notion that public hospitals are relatively inefficient.[8] However, in a 1980 study using different data, Sloan and Steinwald found both total and labor expenses per admission significantly higher in public hospitals than in others.[9]

Case studies by Shonick and colleagues of public systems in 12 urban areas illustrate the effects of transferring the governance of public hospitals from local government to more autonomous agencies formed in conjunction with mergers of public hospitals of public health departments.[10] These mergers and governance changes were not found to be associated with clear gains in operating efficiency.

A related finding concerns contract management of public hospitals by private firms. Several studies indicate that most cost savings and revenue increases generated by a private management firm do not result from greater efficiency (i.e., lowering unit costs) but rather from transferring costs to other public budgets and raising charges paid by patients who are not publicly financed (i.e., cost shifting). In fact, the private companies took little or no direct action to reduce unit costs.[11]

Similarly, a 1986 General Accounting Office (GAO) study of the sale of 40 public hospitals to private ownership found no resulting gains in efficiency. The 40 hospitals had cost increases above the hospital market basket price index. Costs increased mainly due to capital outlays, but administrative expenses also went up. Moreover, the new private owners dramatically increased charges for selected services.[12]

Because of the conflicting evidence, the question of whether a shift to a more autonomous governance structure will increase public hospital efficiency remains open. This issue will be examined in both the case studies and the cross-sectional analysis described below.

*Governance and access.* There is concern that a less publicly accountable, more autonomous governance structure could lead a public hospital to provide less care to the poor and other medically underserved groups. These concerns are based on some of the management practices of for-profit hospitals. "Cream-skimming" policies, which result in restrictions in the number of Medicaid and poor patients treated and reductions in needed but poorly reimbursed services (e.g., alcoholism and drug clinics), have been documented in several areas.[13] For-profit hospitals also treat a disproportionately small number of uninsured patients: an Office for Civil Rights survey showed that only 4 percent of the patient population of for-profit hospitals was uninsured, compared with 37 percent in a sample of large urban public hospitals.[14]

Limited anecdotal evidence also suggests that the practices that for-profit management companies institute in public hospitals could restrict access.[15] Reductions in the availability of outpatient clinic care and the introduction of more aggressive billing and collection procedures have occurred when public hospitals were managed by for-profit firms. The latter practice has caused particular concern to advocates for the underserved, because they believe that for the poor even a small charge is a significant deterrent to seeking health care.[16]

However, a 1982 study of California county hospitals under private management revealed that access restrictions do not always follow more autonomous management.[17] Shonick and Roemer found that levels of services remained unchanged in the public hospitals after private management firms were hired. The number of Medicaid and Medicare patients treated was also substantially unchanged under contract management. The researchers note, however, that discriminatory practices may have been inhibited through close monitoring by the community and the scrutiny of conscientious elected officials. The implication is that the results might have been less positive under different circumstances.

In its 1986 study, the GAO could not obtain sufficient data to document the amount of free care provided by the 40 hospitals before and after the acquisitions.[18] The GAO noted, however, that even though the sale or lease agreements included provisions that the new operators be responsible for indigent care, the hospitals could not document the level of such care they provided, nor were local governments monitoring the level. This implies that access for the indigent was, at a minimum, downplayed after the shift of ownership.

In sum, there is a strong body of opinion suggesting that more autonomous governance will lead a hospital to restrict services to the poor or uninsured, but there is limited evidence either to support or to contradict this hypothesis. The analyses presented in subsequent chapters will test the relationship with both cross-sectional data and time series data for the four case study sites.

*Governance and quality.* Public hospitals are frequently perceived as inferior in quality to other community hospitals. They have been characterized as poorly maintained and underfunded and as the hospitals of last resort. This inferior image stems in part from the hospitals' status as government-run institutions. In a highly market-oriented society, many people associate government control with poor quality that results from a lack of attention to the needs and rights of the individual. Like other large public bureaucracies, a government-run health care provider can be labeled a poorly managed, second-rate institution.

The link between governmental operation and poor quality sometimes goes beyond image; public hospital procedures have been related to poor quality of care. In the 1960s, some of the lower standards of quality of New York City's Department of Hospitals were attributed to fragmented administrative authority, which retarded necessary changes.[19] Many observers claim that civil service regulations keep public hospital administrators from hiring the most highly qualified nonphysician staff and prevent the establishment of incentives for high quality care. It is also alleged that the lack of an incentive to attract private doctors and skilled nurses negatively affects quality of care.[20] Moreover, political involvement is believed to hamper the appointment of skillful and innovative leaders who would encourage the provision of high quality care.

Some observers have argued that a shift to a governing body less closely tied to local government would improve quality of care. Fewer bureaucratic restrictions would result in more responsive decision making, and greater flexibility in staffing would lead to higher quality personnel. More political autonomy would improve the public image of the hospitals and make it possible to attract more privately insured patients who are more likely to voice complaints in order to maintain standards.[21]

There is no systematic empirical evidence to support the widely held belief that governance structure is related to quality of care. In fact, one study dealing with this subject came to an opposite conclusion. Hyman compared the Joint Commission survey reports of municipal and voluntary acute care hospitals in New York City.[22] Municipal hospitals scored better than the voluntaries in the areas of support services and direct medical services. The only area in which the municipal hospitals were judged to have more problems was safety, a component related to physical plant.

In contrast, the GAO study found that the quality of care at hospitals transferred to private ownership improved in terms of physical facilities.[23] In 10 of the 11 transfers studied intensively, the new owners each spent millions of dollars in renovations. They also attempted to improve occupancy rates by recruiting more physicians to practice at the hospital, but occupancy rates did not improve significantly.

The limited available evidence suggests that the general belief that operation by a unit of local government is associated with lower quality than operation by more autonomous forms of governance warrants more careful examination. The case studies presented in this volume include three public systems whose governance structure was changed, in part to improve quality of care. Analysis of their experience should shed some light on the largely unexamined relationship between governance and quality.

**Teaching Affiliation.** Virtually all urban public hospitals have some affiliation with a medical school or teaching hospital. Among the 43 public hospital systems responding to the survey, 42, or fully 98 percent, had some teaching affiliation. Given the almost universal reliance on affiliations by public hospitals, it is informative to examine the "closeness" of these affiliations (see Table 2.2). This can be gauged roughly by considering whether the physicians are employed by the public hospital or the affiliate. Presumably, teaching hospitals that

## Table 2.2

### Employment Arrangements for Residents and for Physician Supervision in Urban Public Hospitals, 1985

| Primary Employer | Supervisory Physicians | | Residents | |
|---|---|---|---|---|
| | Number | Percentage | Number | Percentage |
| Public hospital directly | 15 | 36 | 18 | 43 |
| Contract between physicians and public hospital | 7 | 17 | 3 | 7 |
| Affiliated institution | 11 | 26 | 13 | 31 |
| Public hospital and affiliated institution | 7 | 17 | 7 | 17 |
| Other | 2 | 5 | 1 | 2 |
| Total | 42 | 100 | 42 | 100 |

Source: Authors' survey of public hospitals in 100 largest cities.

assign their own staff to public hospitals or supervise their own staff there are more closely involved than those that only supervise staff who are employees of the public hospital. In 18 of the 42 cities with affiliations, the resident physicians were employed by the public hospital. In another 13 cities the residents were employed by the affiliated medical institution. In the 11 remaining cities, the residents were jointly employed, hired under some contractual arrangement, or employed by a separate foundation.

The employment pattern for supervising physicians was similar. The public hospital was the employer of the supervising staff in 22 of the 42 hospital systems. Of this total, 7 systems had contractual arrangements with the supervising physicians; in the other systems, physicians were employed directly by the public hospital. The affiliated institution employed the supervising physicians in 11 of the cities; in the remaining 9 cities supervising physicians either were employed jointly by both the affiliated institution and the public hospital or had some other distinct arrangement.

Since the vast majority of urban public hospitals are teaching institutions, it also is useful to distinguish among them based on their degree of teaching commitment. One common measure of the size of a hospital's teaching program is its ratio of interns and residents to beds. This measure indicates that urban public teaching hospitals have a greater teaching commitment than their private counterparts. According to the American Hospital Association's annual survey, in 1982 the urban public hospitals had 1.5 residents for every 10 beds compared to less than 0.7 residents for every 10 beds among urban voluntary hospitals. Both public hospitals operated directly by local government and those with more autonomous boards had greater teaching commitments than private hospitals — 1.6 and 1.4, respectively, for every 10 beds.

Although teaching programs appear to be a fact of life for the urban public hospital, their presence is often viewed as a mixed blessing. Public hospitals seek to balance the increased quality expected from the teaching relationship against the increased costs and reduced control over staffing arrangements and service mix that it entails. Public hospitals vary the scale and structure of their teaching affiliations, and those different arrangements are expected to influence the hospitals' efficiency, concern for access, and quality of care.

*Teaching and efficiency.* Teaching programs are expected to generate higher costs per discharge for three reasons. First, length of stay and utilization of ancillary services will be greater because of training needs. Numerous studies have found that interns and residents order more tests and procedures than do fully trained physicians.[24] This is true in both inpatient and outpatient hospital settings.[25]

Second, teaching institutions tend to attract and admit patients with more complex conditions that require more resources for treatment. Finally, teaching hospitals also treat patients with similar conditions more aggressively than do nonteaching hospitals.[26] Some research suggests that these costs of teaching rise as the size of the teaching program increases.[27]

*Teaching and access.* Hospitals with larger teaching programs are believed to provide greater access to care for poor patients, especially for patients without insurance. Indeed, previous research indicates that teaching hospitals provide a significantly greater volume of care to the poor than other hospitals do.[28] Care for the poor is especially high in major teaching hospitals that are members of the Council on Teaching Hospitals (COTH). In 1982, COTH hospitals provided 36 percent of the reported $6.2 billion in bad debt, a significantly higher proportion than their share of charges would indicate.[29] Public teaching hospitals also appear to provide a greater volume of uncompensated care than their voluntary counterparts. Holding other factors constant, public hospitals collectively have uncompensated care case loads 3 percent higher than other hospitals.[30]

Whether urban teaching hospitals provide greater volumes of uncompensated care because of their research and training requirements or simply because they are often located in impoverished areas is not clear. Certainly, a greater commitment to teaching increases the need for "clinical material," which may be supplied by the poor and by those without insurance. On the other hand, the tendency for teaching physicians to be more motivated to treat unusual or rare cases — such as heart or liver transplants — may reduce access to care for uninsured patients who do not meet the specialized interests of research-oriented physicians. Moreover, the outpatient departments of teaching hospitals are generally not organized to provide continuous primary care, an area that full-time faculty have traditionally not viewed as intellectually or financially rewarding. Robb Burlage voiced concern in the 1960s over such negative consequences of teaching affiliations in his review of New York City's policy of developing formal affiliation contracts.[31] The precise contribution of teaching affiliations to the poor's access to care requires further empirical investigation and will be examined in both the case studies and the cross-sectional analyses in this volume.

*Teaching and quality.* Public hospitals with strong teaching affiliations are generally believed to provide higher quality care than they otherwise would be able to provide. Quality enhancements resulting from a strong teaching affiliation include the ability to attract a greater number of talented medical school graduates and the ability to expand and improve services. It is largely because of the expected gains in quality that so many public hospitals, which otherwise find it difficult to recruit physicians, have established teaching relationships. Shonick has written, "It has been a long-standing truism in health services literature that . . . an affiliation with a respected teaching program is a prerequisite for the technological excellence of a public hospital, because much of the medical service in urban public hospitals has been given by house staff supervised by teaching physicians."[32]

Arguments that claim there is a negative relationship between teaching commitments and quality of care point to the tendencies of many teaching institutions to be organized around specialties and to have the provision of tertiary care as their mission. Those characteristics are believed to hinder the efficient and effective organization of primary ambulatory care, an important service component of many public hospitals. The prevalence of multiple specialty clinics in public hospitals and the absence of primary care physicians to coordinate and manage a patient's or even a family's medical care needs is, at least in part, attributed to the traditional teaching orientation of the medical staff in these hospitals.

Affiliation with a medical school has also been shown to be detrimental when the medical service of the public hospital is staffed by medical school physicians who also are affiliated with a medical school hospital. Sparer, in his study of the relationship between the Philadelphia General Hospital and the University of Pennsylvania Medical School, found that financial incentives led physicians to shunt insured patients from the public hospital to the medical school hospital. On many services, the patient census in the public hospital was depleted to such an extent that sufficient standards of quality could not be maintained. Sparer also found that physicians were not actually spending the amount of time at Philadelphia General for which they were being compensated, thus jeopardizing patient access to quality care.[33]

**Financing Arrangements.** Urban public hospitals provide relatively large amounts of care to the indigent. This makes their financing distinct in two respects: they generally receive a significant share of their revenues from local government subsidies, while other hospitals generally do not, and they have a different mix of third-party revenues from that of other hospitals.

Table 2.3 shows the extent to which hospitals with different governing structures vary in their reliance on local government subsidies. Public hospitals covered an average of about 33 percent of their expenses with local subsidies, compared to less than 2 percent for voluntary hospitals. Public hospitals operated as a unit of local government have the highest average tax subsidy, totalling 36 percent of expenses, compared to 29 percent in those public institutions with a separate board.

For revenues derived from third parties, there is an important difference between public and other hospitals. As shown in Table 2.4, the share of revenues from Medicaid was substantially higher than average for public hospitals, accounting for over 17 percent in those public hospitals governed as a unit of local government and nearly one-quarter in the remaining public hospitals, compared to 11 percent in all hospitals. Public hospitals also have significantly less revenue from Medicare and Blue Cross than do other institutions. However, there is little difference in these respects between the two types of public hospital.

*Financing arrangements and efficiency.* Economic theory suggests that greater reliance on local tax subsidies will lead to less efficient operations.[34] Theoretically, incentives to provide a given level and quality of care at minimum cost are reduced when local governments are the payer of last resort. Managers of public hospitals who can "fall back on" a local subsidy are not forced to allocate scarce resources efficiently. As Ellwood and Hoagberg point out, the efficient manager of a public hospital heavily dependent on subsidies may be "rewarded" with reduced appropriations that reflect lower operating costs.[35]

## Table 2.3

## Local Government Subsidy as a Share of
## Total Expenses, 1982

| | Public Hospitals | | | |
| Subsidy | Unit of Government | Separate Board | Total | Voluntary Hospitals |
|---|---|---|---|---|
| Greater than 70% | 0 | 1 | 1 | 0 |
| 51-70% | 2 | 0 | 2 | 1 |
| 26-50% | 3 | 4 | 7 | 0 |
| 10-25% | 2 | 4 | 6 | 1 |
| Less than 10% | 2 | 1 | 3 | 51 |
| Total | 9 | 10 | 19 | 53 |
| Mean percentage of expenses | 36% | 29% | 33% | 2% |

Source: "Survey of Medical Care for the Poor and Hospitals' Financial Status, 1982" (joint survey of the American Hospital Association and the Urban Institute; hereafter cited as 1982 joint AHA-Urban Institute survey).

Note: Data are shown only for hospitals reporting a local subsidy. For most public hospitals not reporting, the figure was not reported in the survey; for most voluntary hospitals not reporting, the figure is probably zero.

## Table 2.4

## Revenue from Major Third-Party Payers,
## Hospitals in 100 Largest Cities, 1982

| | Percentage of Hospital's Total Revenue | | | | |
| Type of Hospital | Medicaid | Medicare | Blue Cross | Commercial | Self-Pay |
|---|---|---|---|---|---|
| Public — unit of local government | 17.4 | 22.8 | 6.4 | 11.1 | 5.9 |
| Public — separate board | 24.4 | 21.1 | 8.1 | 8.8 | 6.5 |
| Private nonprofit | 10.9 | 31.8 | 18.2 | 25.0 | 5.2 |
| For-profit | 8.0 | 33.6 | 12.3 | 38.6 | 2.8 |
| All hospitals combined | 11.4 | 31.2 | 17.2 | 24.3 | 5.2 |

Source: 1982 joint AHA-Urban Institute survey.

The available research on this issue is limited and does not support the economic theory. A study of California hospitals found that county-owned hospitals, which rely on local subsidies, had unit costs 5 percent below the average California hospital—8 percent lower when adjusted for case mix.[36] Broader studies of unit costs at hospitals with different governance and finance arrangements have not been completed, but evidence on this subject will be presented in the cross-sectional analysis and case studies of this book.

*Financing arrangements and access.* The links between financing arrangements and access for the poor parallel the conceptual links between governance and access. Strong ties to local government, including a heavy dependence on local tax subsidies, are likely to increase pressures for service to the indigent. Thus, more heavily subsidized hospitals can be expected to provide more services to the uninsured poor. There are no systematic comparative data on local subsidies, but this relationship will be explored in the four case studies.

*Financing arrangements and quality.* The previously described hypothetical links between governance structure and quality are also believed to underlie a causal connection between local subsidies and quality of care. That is, local subsidies are believed to be an unreliable source of revenue, and the associated fiscal uncertainties are alleged to cause lower quality care. Local subsidies are also believed to favor operating over capital expenses, causing heavily subsidized public systems to have more deteriorated physical plants. The tendency of local governments to underinvest in capital affects quality by making acquisition of modern equipment difficult and by resulting in neglected or aged physical plants that are not attractive to patients, that hinder recruitment of staff, and that make delivery of sophisticated care more difficult.

With respect to uncertainty, local subsidies are reported to vary widely from year to year depending on local political and fiscal conditions and to be subject to modifications for unanticipated reasons even during the course of a year. Such variations and modifications make well-planned and adequate staffing difficult and may hinder the recruitment and retention of well-qualified personnel.

As noted in the discussion of governance and quality, there is little or no empirical evidence establishing relationships between quality of care and aspects of hospital governance and financing. This relationship will be explored in the case studies.

**Marketing Strategy.** The procompetition philosophy of the Reagan administration has encouraged many hospitals to engage in competitive marketing activities. Although presented as a strategy to control health care costs and enhance consumers' freedom of choice, the promotion of competition and marketing activities may also exacerbate the problems of urban public hospitals. It is argued that these institutions, with their higher unit costs and large volume of uncompensated care, will be at a disadvantage in a competitive system.[37] Nevertheless, some public hospitals are emulating private hospitals in pursuing such marketing strategies as service differentiation and market segmentation. These hospitals typically emphasize generously reimbursed, tertiary care services. Other urban public hospitals have chosen to emphasize primary care services to low-income populations. These institutions pursue a strategy of "vertical integration": the hospital is linked to freestanding ambulatory care centers and to long-term care facilities affording access to the poor and uninsured. The Denver system, a merger of the local public hospital and the local public health department, is the best-known and most successful example of this strategy. Prior research and the observations of health care analysts suggest that the strategy chosen will affect efficiency, access, and quality of care.

*Marketing strategy and efficiency.* Advocates of competition believe that competition will lead to decreased costs, at least in the long run. Available research does not support this contention, however. Becker and Sloan compared cost and profitability among for-profit, private nonprofit, and public hospitals. Although the marketing strategies of the hospitals were not specifically identified, for-profit hospitals were generally characterized by more competitive behavior. The evidence indicated no difference in unit costs, after controlling for other factors, between for-profit and other types of hospitals.[38] The study did show, however, that a more complex service mix and a higher proportion of privately insured patients were related to hospital profitability. This suggests that a strategy of attracting more insured patients and emphasizing more generously reimbursed services may improve "bottom line" results but not true economic efficiency. In fact, a market orientation could lead to increased unit costs. The newer facilities, enhanced amenities, and increased staffing needed to compete effectively could drive up unit costs.

*Marketing strategy and access.* A competitive market stance may adversely affect a public hospital's provision of care to the poor in two ways. First, and perhaps less likely, medically indigent patients could be crowded out if the hospital is highly successful in changing its image and attracts a large number of privately insured patients. Second, services that are heavily utilized by the poor, such as emergency rooms and outpatient clinics, could be cut back because of management decisions to eliminate or minimize unprofitable services. The anecdotal evidence noted earlier about the strategies pursued by private contract management firms makes this a potential concern.

*Marketing strategy and quality.* The potential connection between market strategies and quality of care is only indirect. To the extent that public hospitals seeking to compete for privately insured patients are successful, their quality of care may be improved, because privately insured paying patients are believed to be more demanding of adequate levels of service and more effective in voicing their demands. Another indirect consequence of a successful strategy to increase privately insured patients could be higher operating margins and hence more resources to improve physical plants and enhance staffing.

The connections between marketing strategy and each of the three performance criteria have not been studied carefully, because only recently have there emerged any significant number of urban public hospitals adopting a more competitive strategy and because of the close association between policy decisions regarding market strategy and policy decisions relating to financing and governance arrangements.

## Relations among Policy Variables

As the discussion of marketing strategies indicated, there is likely to be a pattern of relationships among some of the policy variables. Financing arrangements, governance structure, and marketing strategy are likely to cluster in certain patterns. One expected pattern is that heavy dependence on local subsidies will be associated with more direct political control by the unit of local government, a pattern that will lead to very limited efforts by the hospital to engage in competition for private patients. A related expectation is that changes in governance leading to more political autonomy for the hospital will be associated with efforts to reduce local subsidies and may facilitate policies to increase the number of privately insured patients served by the hospital.

The relationships between degree of teaching commitment and other policy variables are less clear. On the one hand, more autonomous and more competitive public hospitals may seek to strengthen their teaching missions because this will expand their specialized or tertiary services and thereby enhance their attractiveness as referral centers for privately insured patients. Alternatively, more autonomous and competitive public hospitals might seek only limited teaching affiliations in order to reduce reliance on salaried medical staff and provide greater opportunities for community physicians in private practice to admit their insured patients. Reduced teaching commitments might also reduce unit costs and make the hospital more price-competitive.

In summary, there are many unanswered questions about the nature of the policy decisions that structure urban public hospitals and about the links between those policies and the performance criteria of efficiency, access, and quality. This study uses two different research strategies to clarify these relationships and to test some specific hypotheses.

## Research Methods

In the social sciences, empirical research is generally designed to test hypotheses. The hypotheses are deduced from theory or developed inductively. The previous section revealed, however, that the relationships between the policy decisions affecting local public hospitals and the hospitals' performance are complex and not very conducive to testing. Although there are theoretically derived hypotheses linking, for example, governance status and efficiency, there also are relationships for which theory provides no guidance and for which inductive reasoning yields contradicting hypotheses. For example, the case has been made that competitive market strategies could both reduce the poor's access to care by making uninsured patients less attractive and increase the poor's access to care by providing greater opportunities for "successful" hospitals to shift costs to help finance the care of the uninsured (at least in the short run).

Given the varied state of theory and hypothesis development relating to the performance of public hospitals, two research tasks can be identified. First, there are some relatively well-developed hypotheses that can be investigated through quasi-experimental designs. Specifically, the following hypotheses can be tested:

1. Greater autonomy in the governance of a public hospital system (i.e., the establishment of semi-independent boards) will lead to both greater efficiency (i.e., lower unit costs) and reduced access to care for the poor (i.e., lower volume of Medicaid and uncompensated care).

2. More intensive teaching relationships at public hospitals (i.e., a higher ratio of interns and residents to beds) will lead to both reduced efficiency (i.e., higher unit costs) and greater access to care for the poor.

In addition to those hypotheses, there are several relationships both among the policy variables themselves and between policy variables and performance measures that require greater understanding. For example, how closely linked are governance and financing relationships and how do they affect quality?

To accomplish the dual tasks of relatively rigorous testing of well-defined hypotheses and of exploratory research to improve our understanding of relationships in order to formulate more refined hypotheses, two different research methods are required. The cross-sectional analysis used for hypothesis testing is described briefly below and more fully in Chapter 7; the remaining sections of this chapter present the case method approach and case study sites.

## Cross-Sectional Analysis

Cross-sectional analysis using multiple regression techniques has become a widely accepted approach to hypothesis testing in the social sciences. However, the valid use of this approach requires quantitative measures of the relevant variables and available data for these measures for a relatively large sample. These prerequisites were met for the hypotheses presented above, largely with data from a joint American Hospital Association–Urban Institute survey of hospitals conducted in 1982. From this survey, a data set was constructed that included quantitative measures of the performance criteria of access and efficiency, of the policy variables of governance and teaching commitment, and of several relevant control variables. Chapter 7 describes the data sources and the regression equations more completely.

## Case Study Analysis

Case studies are particularly well suited to the research task of developing an understanding of processes and thereby formulating more sophisticated hypotheses. Since the ways in which governance, financing, marketing, and teaching policies influence public hospital performance are not well understood, a set of case studies should provide opportunities to broaden such knowledge. Accordingly, case studies of changes in four large public hospital systems were completed—the Health and Hospitals Corporation in New York City, the Los Angeles County Hospitals Department, the Hillsborough County Hospital Authority in Florida's Hillsborough County, and the Regional Medical Center at Memphis in Shelby County, Tennessee.

The case studies focus on the five-year period 1980–84 and present relevant historical background material. Each case emphasizes how the policy decisions regarding governance structure, finance arrangements, teaching relationships, and market strategy affect the performance criteria of efficiency, access, and quality. When, during the study period, any of the policy variables was changed significantly (e.g., a change in governance structure), special attention was given to the consequences of the change.

In completing the case studies, three major types of data were used—interviews, primary documents, and secondary sources. Persons interviewed included local government representatives responsible for oversight of the public hospital, hospital board members, chief executive and fiscal officers of the hospital, and others knowledgeable about the public and private hospital systems in the community. A formal interview protocol was prepared and used for most interviews. In New York City, however, the mayor's office did not grant permission for formal interviews, so those interviews were less systematic and less formal. However, the research staff met with numerous public hospital and city government officials during the course of the study.

The primary documents used in the study included the audited financial reports and other annual reports for the study hospitals, internal reports on utilization for the hospitals, Joint Commission reports (or summaries thereof) for the hospitals, consultant and other special reports prepared for the hospitals, and local government agency reports on the hospitals. Secondary sources included published works on the local area health systems and newspaper and other media reports on the study hospitals.

**Case Study Sites.** The selection of case study sites involved addressing two questions: How many cases should be analyzed? By what criteria should the cases be selected?

The issue of how many cases was somewhat arbitrarily decided by a combination of resource constraints and common sense. Clearly, more than one or two cases were desirable to avoid highly idiosyncratic results. The decision to select four sites was based in part on the belief that in-depth analysis would serve the heuristic purposes better than more numerous but less intensive investigations. It was also a sufficient number to encompass substantial variation in the key policy variables.

The specific sites were selected based on a combination of the size of the sites and the variation in their governance structures and market strategies. The nation's two largest local public hospital systems—New York and Los Angeles—are of special interest because of their large size and their importance in their communities. In addition, the New York system is governed by a semiautonomous board while the Los Angeles system remains within county government. The Tampa and Memphis systems are large and important systems that are pursuing competitive market strategies, and each recently changed governance structure partly in connection with these new strategies.

*Policy variables.* The variations in policy characteristics among the selected sites are summarized in Table 2.5. Three of the four sites (all but Los Angeles) are governed by semi-independent boards. However, New

## Table 2.5
## Policy Characteristics of Case Study Hospital Systems

|  | New York City | Los Angeles County | Hillsborough County | Shelby County |
|---|---|---|---|---|
| Governance—legal structure | Semi-independent board since 1970 | Unit of local government since creation | Semi-independent board since 1980 | Semi-independent board since 1981 |
| Teaching—residents per bed | .301 | .418 | .170 | .310 |
| Financing—expenses covered by local government subsidy | 24% | 27% | 5% | 33% |
| Market strategy—discharges covered by private insurance (including Blue Cross) | 12% | 8% | 33% | 46% |

York has had such governance arrangements since 1970, whereas Tampa shifted from a unit of local government in 1980 and Memphis did so in 1981. In the two latter sites, the case study period spans the time of transition.

The public hospitals vary in their financing arrangements and particularly in their reliance on local government subsidies. During the latest year for which data were available, three of the hospitals depended on such subsidies for about one-quarter to one-third of their operating revenues. In contrast, the Tampa hospital had reduced its subsidy share to about 5 percent. In each case the figure varied annually, and the consequences of these changes in level of local subsidy are considered in the analysis. In addition, each of the hospitals received a significant share of its revenues from Medicaid, and the links between this largely state-determined financing program and hospital performance were also considered.

Each of the study hospitals had significant teaching programs, but the degree of teaching varied. The ratio of residents to beds was highest in Los Angeles and lowest in Tampa; New York's ratio was similar to that in Memphis. Although none of the hospitals implemented substantial changes in its teaching programs during the study period, the considerable variation in teaching commitment permits some inferences to be drawn by comparing sites.

Finally, the case study hospitals are divided evenly between those actively pursuing relatively competitive market strategies and those committed primarily to serving the indigent. Both New York and Los Angeles have relatively small shares of privately insured patients and are not actively engaged in programs to change substantially the economic mix of their patients. In contrast, Tampa and Memphis launched significant efforts to increase their numbers and shares of privately insured patients during the study period, and they are characterized by larger percentages of inpatient services to these patients.

*Other characteristics of study sites.* As background for the case studies it is useful to be aware not only of the configuration of policy variables but also of how they vary with respect to the characteristics of the populations of the areas in which the hospitals are located and the characteristics of the broader community health care systems in which the hospitals operate. Tables 2.6 through 2.8 present data describing those features of the case study sites.

The four sites varied in population size from Hillsborough County's (Tampa) 647,000 people to Los Angeles County's nearly 7.5 million people. The population in New York City was declining; in Los Angeles County and Shelby County (Memphis) it was growing at rates below the

## Table 2.6

## Population Characteristics of Case Study Sites, 1980

| | New York City | Los Angeles County | Hillsborough County | Shelby County | U.S. |
|---|---|---|---|---|---|
| Total population | | | | | |
| People | 7,071,639 | 7,477,503 | 646,960 | 777,113 | 226,545,805 |
| Households | 2,788,221 | 2,730,674 | 237,943 | 269,186 | 82,227,411 |
| Percent change in number of people since 1970 | (10.4%) | 6.3% | 32.0% | 7.6% | 11.5% |
| Composition by sex (percent) | | | | | |
| Male | 46.3% | 48.8% | 48.3% | 47.8% | 48.6% |
| Female | 53.7 | 51.2 | 51.7 | 52.2 | 51.4 |
| Black and Hispanic population (percent) | | | | | |
| Black | 25.3% | 12.6% | 13.4% | 41.7% | 11.7% |
| Hispanic | 19.9 | 27.6 | 9.9 | 0.9 | 6.5 |
| Composition by age (percent) | | | | | |
| 14 years and younger | 20.7% | 22.0% | 21.8% | 24.0% | 22.6% |
| 15–54 years old | 56.0 | 58.7 | 57.2 | 58.1 | 59.5 |
| 55 years and older | 24.1 | 19.3 | 21.1 | 17.8 | 20.9 |
| Income | | | | | |
| Median family income | $19,268 | $21,135 | $17,697 | $18,193 | $19,917 |
| Proportion of population below poverty (percent) | 19.7% | 13.2% | 13.8% | 19.0% | 12.1% |

Source: Arca Resource File, Office of Data Analysis and Management, Bureau of Health Professions, U.S. Department of Health and Human Services.

## Table 2.7

## Health Status Characteristics of Case Study Sites, 1980

| | New York City | Los Angeles County | Hillsborough County | Shelby County | U.S. |
|---|---|---|---|---|---|
| Births per 1,000 population | 14.5 | 17.8 | 15.1 | 18.3 | 15.9 |
| Proportion of births to women under 20 | 17.7% | 7.0% | 19.5% | 19.9% | 15.4% |
| Deaths per 100,000 population | | | | | |
| All causes | 1,061 | 821 | 891 | 890 | 880 |
| Infectious disease | 8 | 6 | 7 | 9 | 8 |
| Malignancies | 222 | 169 | 196 | 188 | 184 |
| Ischemic heart disease | 438 | 194 | 216 | 177 | 250 |
| Cardiovascular disease | 135 | 215 | 195 | 252 | 187 |
| Influenza | 45 | 24 | 26 | 21 | 24 |
| Bronchitis | 20 | 22 | 32 | 24 | 25 |
| Cirrhosis | 30 | 20 | 16 | 11 | 14 |
| Motor vehicle accident | 11 | 20 | 28 | 21 | 23 |
| Other causes | 152 | 151 | 175 | 187 | 165 |
| Infant deaths per 1,000 births | | | | | |
| 1980 | 15.0 | 11.9 | 16.5 | 16.3 | 12.6 |
| 1974–78 | 17.5 | 13.6 | 15.7 | 17.4 | 15.2 |
| White, 1974–78 | 14.4 | 12.3 | 12.8 | 13.7 | 13.3 |
| Nonwhite, 1974–78 | 22.7 | 18.4 | 25.7 | 20.7 | 23.0 |

Source: See Table 2.6.

# Table 2.8

## Health Services Supply and Utilization Characteristics of Case Study Sites

| | New York City | Los Angeles County | Hillsborough County | Shelby County | U.S. |
|---|---|---|---|---|---|
| Active MDs (1982) | | | | | |
| Total number | 25,286 | 19,956 | 1,358 | 3,099 | 438,916 |
| Number per 1,000 population | 3.58 | 2.67 | 2.10 | 2.70 | 1.94 |
| Patient care MDs (1981) | | | | | |
| Total number | 21,101 | 17,619 | 1,171 | 1,870 | 389,468 |
| Number per 1,000 population | 2.98 | 2.36 | 1.81 | 2.40 | 1.68 |
| Office-based MDs (1981) | | | | | |
| Total number | 11,736 | 13,592 | 877 | 1,205 | 284,313 |
| Number per 1,000 population | 1.66 | 1.82 | 1.36 | 1.55 | 1.24 |
| Short-term general hospitals | | | | | |
| Number of hospitals, 1983 | 70 | 141 | 13 | 11 | 5,959 |
| Hospital beds, 1980 | 34,541 | 32,721 | 2,869 | 6,154 | 952,867 |
| Beds per 1,000 population, 1980 | 4.88 | 4.38 | 4.43 | 7.92 | 3.57 |
| Hospital admissions, 1982 | 1,129,099 | 1,086,755 | 122,871 | 186,104 | 37,424,647 |
| Admissions per 1,000 population, 1982 | 159.66 | 145.34 | 189.92 | 239.48 | 165.19 |
| Acute care inpatient days,1983 | 7,143,059 | 5,583,862 | 774,630 | 1,076,763 | 206,882,702 |
| Days per 1,000 population, 1983 | 1,010.10 | 746.76 | 1,197.33 | 1,385.59 | 913.20 |

Source: See Table 2.6.

national average; and in Hillsborough County it grew by about one-third in the 1970s, a rate nearly triple the national average.

Although generally similar and close to national averages in the sex compositions of their populations, the four sites varied in ethnic and age compositions. The black population ranged from only slightly above the national average in Los Angeles County and Hillsborough County to over one-quarter in New York City and fully 42 percent in Shelby County. The Hispanic population ranged from less than 1 percent of the total population in Shelby County to nearly 28 percent in Los Angeles County. Thus, all of the areas had a substantial population of some ethnic minority, although the mix varied. In addition, all of the sites had a proportion of people living in poverty that was larger than the national average.

The age distribution of the cities' populations varied notably. Both Hillsborough County and New York City were relatively old, with low proportions of young people and high proportions of the elderly. In contrast, Los Angeles County and Shelby County had relatively few elderly residents and more younger residents.

The diverse ethnic and age characteristics of the populations were related to varied health conditions and problems in the study sites (see Table 2.7). Birthrates were above the national average in Shelby and Los Angeles counties, largely because of their younger population. The two southern counties had higher rates of births to teenage mothers, while Los Angeles's teenage birthrate was less than half the national average.

The mortality rate in Los Angeles County was also significantly below the national average. The lower rate of deaths from ischemic heart disease was the main factor. New York City, in contrast, had a mortality rate more than 20 percent above the national average, primarily because of higher death rates from malignancies and ischemic heart disease. Hillsborough and Shelby counties had mortality rates only slightly higher than the national average.

Infant mortality, like overall mortality and teenage birthrate, was lowest and below the national average in Los Angeles County. In contrast, infant mortality was well above the national average in the other three sites. In all of the sites infant mortality was significantly higher for minorities than for whites. However, only in Hillsborough County was nonwhite infant mortality above that group's national average.

The health care systems providing services in each of the four study sites were characterized by relatively generous resources. The ratio of patient care physicians to population was well above the national average in all four sites as was the ratio of hospital beds to population. However, there was significant variation among the sites on these indicators, with patient care physicians per 1,000 population ranging from 1.81 in Hillsborough County to 2.98 in New York City and hospital beds per 1,000 population ranging from 4.38 in Los Angeles County to 7.92 in Shelby County.

Despite the relatively generous supply of hospital beds in all sites, there was significant variation in use of hospital inpatient services. Admission rates were below the national average in both New York City and Los Angeles County; however, relatively short lengths of stay in Los Angeles County kept total days per 1,000 population well below the national average, while relatively long lengths of stay in New York City pushed total days per 1,000 population well above the national average. The relatively high admission rates in Hillsborough and Shelby counties were not offset by short lengths of stay, resulting in rates of hospital days per 1,000 population well above the national average.

## Conclusion

This volume seeks to determine whether and how local policy decisions regarding the governance, financing, and staffing of public hospitals affect the performance of those hospitals. A review of the literature on this subject reveals little well-established knowledge on these issues, a few well-formulated hypotheses, and much uncertainty about many causal connections.

To advance the state of knowledge on these issues, this study presents empirical evidence to test selected hypotheses that link governance structures and teaching relationships to public hospital performance. In addition, a set of four case studies will be presented as a source of deeper understanding of the relationships among policy variables and the ways in which they influence public hospital performance. The four case studies — New York, Los Angeles, Tampa, and Memphis — represent large urban public hospitals that have differing client populations and operate in diverse health care delivery systems.

## Notes

1. *Accreditation Manual for Hospitals, 1983* (Chicago: Joint Commission on Accreditation of Hospitals, 1982).
2. See, for example, Harold Demsetz, "Some Aspects of Property Rights," *Journal of Law and Economics* 61 (April 1966): 1–22; and Louis De Alissi, "The Economics of Property Rights: A Review of the Evidence," *American Economic Review* 73, no. 1 (March 1983): 64–81.
3. Kenneth Clarkson, "Some Implications of Property Rights in Hospital

Management," *Journal of Law and Economics* 23, no. 2 (October 1972): 363–84; and E. Becker and F. Sloan, "Hospital Ownership and Performance," *Economic Inquiry* 23 (January 1985): 21–36.

4. Mark Pauly and Michael Redisch, "The Not for Profit Hospital as a Physician's Cooperative," *American Economic Review* 63 (March 1973): 87–99.

5. W. A. Niskanen, *Bureaucracy and Representative Government* (Chicago: Aldene Publishers, 1971).

6. Charles Wolf, Jr., "A Theory of Nonmarket Failure: Framework for Implementation Analysis," *Journal of Law and Economics* 22, no. 1 (April 1979): 107–40.

7. Becker and Sloan, "Hospital Ownership and Performance."

8. Samuel Wolfe and H. Sherer, *Public General Hospitals in Crisis* (Washington, DC: Coalition of American Public Employees, 1977).

9. Frank Sloan and Bruce Steinwald, *Insurance Regulation and Hospital Costs* (Lexington, MA: D.C. Heath, 1980).

10. William Shonick, "Mergers of Public Health Departments with Public Hospitals in Urban Areas: Findings of 12 Field Studies," *Medical Care*, supplement (August 1980); and William Shonick and Walter Price, "Reorganization of Health Agencies by Local Government in American Urban Centers: What Do They Portend for 'Public Health'?" *Milbank Memorial Fund Quarterly* 55, no. 2 (Spring 1977): 233–71.

11. "Contract Management: Report on the 1980 Survey of Contract Managed Hospitals and Three Case Studies," in *Studies in the Comparative Performance of Investor-Owned and Not-for-Profit Hospitals*, vol. 2 (Washington, DC: Lewin and Associates, 1981); and W. Shonick and R. Roemer, *Public Hospitals Under Private Management: The California Experience* (Berkeley, CA: Institute of Governmental Studies, University of California, 1983).

12. General Accounting Office, *Public Hospital Sales Lead to Better Facilities but Increased Patient Costs*, Human Resources Division 86-60 (Washington, DC: U.S. Government Printing Office, June 1986).

13. See Mareasa R. Isaacs, K. G. Litchner, and C. M. Lipschultz, *The Urban Public Hospital: Options for the 1980s* (Bethesda, MD: Alpha Center, 1982), pp. 133–35.

14. Survey data cited in Isaacs, Litchner, and Lipschultz, *The Urban Public Hospital*, p. 134.

15. Isaacs, Litchner, and Lipschultz, *The Urban Public Hospital*.

16. G. Dallek, ed., *The Struggle to Save Public Hospitals: An Advocacy Guide* (Los Angeles: National Health Law Program, 1981).

17. Shonick and Roemer, *Public Hospitals Under Private Management*.

18. General Accounting Office, *Public Hospital Sales*.

19. *Community Health Services for New York City: Report and Staff Studies of the Commission on the Delivery of Personal Health Services* (New York: Praeger Publishers, 1969).

20. For example, see L. Breslow, "Role of the Public Hospital," *Hospitals* 44, no. 13 (1 July 1970): 44–46; and Alice Tetelman, "Public Hospitals: Critical or Recovering?" *Health Services Reports* 88, no. 4 (1973): 295–304.

21. This argument is made in Karin Dumbaugh, J. Bent, and D. Nauhauser, "Public Hospitals: An Evaluation," *Academy of Political Science Proceedings* 32, no. 3 (1977): 148–58.

22. Herbert Hyman, "Are Public Hospitals in New York City Inferior to Vol-

untary Nonprofit Hospitals? A Study of JCAH Hospital Surveys," *American Journal of Public Health* 76, no. 1 (January 1985): 18-22.
23. General Accounting Office, *Public Hospital Sales*.
24. E. W. Martz and R. Ptakowski, "Educational Costs to Hospitalized Patients," *Journal of Medical Education* 53, no. 5 (1978): 383-86; and J. M. Eisenberg and D. Nicklin, "Use of Diagnostic Services by Physicians in Community Practice," *Medical Care* 19, no. 3 (1981): 297-309.
25. B. Schultz, "An Analysis of Hospital Ambulatory Care Costs" (Ph.D. diss., New York University, 1975).
26. A. Garber, V. Fuchs, and J. Silverman, "Casemix, Costs and Outcomes: Differences Between Faculty and Community Services in a University Hospital," *New England Journal of Medicine* 310, no. 19 (18 July 1985): 157-62.
27. K. Thorpe, S. Cretin, and E. Keeler, *Are the DRG Weights Compressed?* (Santa Monica, CA: Rand Corporation, 1986).
28. Judith Feder, Jack Hadley, and Ross Mullner, "Falling Through the Cracks: Poverty, Insurance Coverage, and Hospital Care to the Poor, 1980 and 1982," *Milbank Memorial Fund Quarterly* 62, no. 4 (Fall 1984): 544-66; and Frank Sloan, Joseph Valvona, and Ross Mullner, "Identifying the Issues: A Statistical Profile," in Frank Sloan, Joseph Valvona, and Ross Mullner, eds., *Uncompensated Hospital Care, Rights and Responsibilities* (Baltimore: Johns Hopkins University Press, 1986).
29. Sloan, Valvona, and Mullner, "Identifying the Issues."
30. Ibid.
31. Robb K. Burlage, *New York City's Municipal Hospitals: A Policy Review* (Washington, DC: Institute for Policy Studies, 1967).
32. William Shonick, "Early Developments and Recent Trends in the Evolution of the Local Public Hospital," *Annual Review of Public Health* 5 (1984): 53.
33. Edward V. Sparer, *Medical School Accountability in the Public Hospital: The University of Pennsylvania Medical School and the Philadelphia General Hospital* (Philadelphia: Health Law Project, 1974).
34. Harvey Liebenstein, "Aspects of the X-Efficiency Theory of the Firm," *Bell Journal of Economics* 6, no. 2 (Autumn 1975): 580-606.
35. Paul M. Ellwood, Jr., and E. J. Hoagberg, "Problems of Public Hospitals," *Hospitals* 44, no. 13 (1 July 1970): 47-52.
36. This study is cited in E. R. Brown, "Public Hospitals on the Brink: Their Problems and Their Options," *Journal of Health Politics, Policy and Law* 7, no. 4 (Winter 1983): 927-44.
37. Isaacs, Litchner, and Lipschultz, *The Urban Public Hospital*.
38. Becker and Sloan, "Hospital Ownership and Performance."

# ᘓ 3 ᘔ

# New York City Health and Hospitals Corporation

## Charles Brecher, Kenneth E. Thorpe, and Cynthia Green

The network of facilities operated by the New York City Health and Hospitals Corporation (HHC) constitutes the largest and most expensive local public hospital system in the United States. Its continued operation and high level of funding—total expenditures of nearly $2 billion including over $400 million of local tax funds—evidence a local political commitment to ensuring accessible medical care for New Yorkers regardless of income. This case study describes the governance, financing, market strategy, and medical staffing arrangements established by the city and state of New York for the HHC. It also identifies the relationships between these policy decisions and the HHC's performance with respect to ensuring access to care and the provision of high quality services.

The first section of this chapter provides essential background on the history of New York City's municipal hospital system and on the regulatory climate established by the state of New York. The second section reviews the recent performance of the HHC on indicators of efficiency, quality, and access to care for the local indigent population. The next four sections focus, respectively, on the policy decisions determining the governance structure, financing arrangements, medical staffing, and market strategy for the HHC. In each case the nature of the current arrangements is described and their effects on efficiency, quality, and access are analyzed. The final section distills the lessons of the New York City experience.

## Background

Current arrangements for New York City's municipal hospitals have evolved as responses to changing conditions in the city and changing federal and state policies for financing and delivering health care. To understand the implications of the current situation for the quality and efficiency of care and access to care, it is useful to review the historical circumstances leading to current policies.

### Organizational History

Historically, New York City's provision of medical care to needy individuals through municipally operated institutions has been a source of pride as well as a target of reform.[1] In the nineteenth century the city provided medical care for poor individuals at infirmaries attached to its poorhouses, and these facilities evolved into separate hospitals. In 1929, responsibility for operating these facilities was shifted from the welfare department to a newly created hospitals department.

During the Depression the scale of operation expanded to meet a growing need as an estimated 60 percent of the city's population was eligible for care at public expense under then-prevailing rules. Municipal hospitals became overcrowded, and the city launched a major program of purchasing hospital care for indigents from underutilized voluntary hospitals. At prices less than the full cost of care, the city eventually purchased care for about one-third of its total indigent patient load from voluntary hospitals in addition to operating a large municipal hospital system at nearly 100 percent occupancy.

During the Depression, the reform administration of Mayor Fiorello LaGuardia, under the leadership of Hospitals Commissioner F. S. Goldwater, instituted a number of changes designed primarily to remove political patronage and corrupt practices from the hospitals department. Employees were placed under the civil service system, purchases of supplies and letting of contracts became subject to careful review and centralized standards, and the Bureau of the Budget, created in 1933, was given authority to monitor expenditures. Physicians, underemployed during the Depression, were recruited on a paid, part-time basis for outpatient clinics and donated their time for inpatient care. Additional physician staff were secured for three hospitals through affiliation arrangements. Bellevue, long a teaching site for the city's leading medical schools, had supervising physicians from Columbia University and New York University; later, in 1939, limited affiliations were initiated between Kings County Hospital and the Long Island College of Medicine and between Metropolitan Hospital and New York Medical College. If the New York City municipal hospitals ever had a "good old days" period it was the decade preceding World War II, when they served a large proportion of the population under administrative and medical care arrangements that were perceived as steadily improving, if not fully satisfactory.

**The Post-World War II Decline.** The 15 years following World War II witnessed a decline in the standing of the municipal hospital system. Four major factors underlay this decline. First, the physical plant deteriorated seriously. Inadequate and overutilized even before the war, municipal facilities received little new investment during the Depression and war years. Some new capital investment was made after the war, but it was directed primarily at building new hospitals. Between 1950 and 1960, the city opened new facilities at the Bronx Municipal Hospital Center, Coney Island Hospital in Brooklyn, Elmhurst Hospital in Queens, and Metropolitan Hospital in Manhattan. The rest of the system, however, was neglected. Ancient facilities, such as the pre-1900 Lincoln Hospital building, were not adequately cared for or replaced. This same period was one of major construction for the voluntary sector, which benefited from federal construction funds to help rebuild and expand its plant. Thus a growing disparity developed between the quality of facilities in the two sectors.

Second, economic and technological forces were working to reduce demand for municipal hospital services while making hospital care a more expensive product. Group hospital insurance for the working population became widespread during this period, reducing demand for municipal hospital services and increasing occupancy at the newer voluntary facilities. Improvements in the nature of medical care made it a more expensive service as its technological component grew. Standards of nursing care and the need for technical manpower increased, making hospitals more expensive to staff.

Municipal appropriations for hospitals did not keep pace with these cost pressures, which led to a perception that the municipal hospitals were underfunded. Equipment was not always modern. Staffing was often inadequate, particularly for nursing and other technical positions that could not be filled at permitted salaries; as a result, municipal hospitals came to rely on less-skilled employees.

Part of the explanation for the city's budgetary pressure was that demands from the voluntary sector were escalating for payments for the services it provided to the poor — even as the city's own hospitals experienced declining occupancy. In fiscal year 1961, for example, the city spent $38 million for the voluntary hospitals and $176 million for the municipal hospitals.[2]

Third, changes in physician education and supply made it increasingly difficult for the municipal facilities to recruit and maintain adequate physician staff. Because of the American Medical Association's control over medical school capacity, the nation's physician supply did not keep pace with population growth. Given a wider range of choices than they had had during the Depression, doctors in the immediate postwar era generally chose to serve middle-class patients with health insurance. Physicians remaining on the staff of the public hospitals tended to be older men with practices located in poorer neighborhoods. Younger and better-trained doctors followed their more affluent patients to the suburbs. By the end of the 1950s most of the municipal hospitals were relying heavily on foreign-trained doctors for staff, several institutions were threatened with loss of accreditation because of inadequate staff, and one hospital — Gouverneur — was obliged to close in 1959.

Finally, the administrative reforms of the LaGuardia era came to be perceived as bureaucratic obstacles to efficient management in the new period of more technologically sophisticated medical care. Centralized control over the budget, civil service procedures, and purchasing regulations led to rigidities in the operation of the municipal hospitals. The combination of old and poorly maintained facilities, underfunding for operations, a shortage of medical staff, and inappropriate administrative controls led to a serious deterioration in the quality of services available at municipal hospitals in the postwar era.

**Establishment of the Affiliation System.** The deterioration in the level of service at municipal hospitals eventually led to strong political pressures to take remedial action.[3] In February of 1959, Mayor Robert F. Wagner appointed a blue-ribbon commission on health services, chaired by David Heyman, an investment banker active in creating the Health Insurance Plan of Greater New York. The Heyman Commission report in July of 1960 was followed six months later by a similar effort sponsored by the Hospital Council of Greater New York. While the two commission reports differed in their emphases, both highlighted the staff problems of the municipal hospitals and identified closer relations with medical schools and voluntary teaching hospitals as a partial solution.

The commission reports alone did not lead to action, but they identified a path to be followed when crisis struck. The crisis arrived early in 1961, following the failure of Gouverneur Hospital to achieve accreditation and the failure of most of the house staff at Harlem Hospital to pass the mandatory examinations for foreign medical graduates initiated in that year. To cope with the situation, Mayor Wagner appointed a new hospitals commissioner, Dr. Ray Trussel from Columbia University's medical center, and gave him a mandate to develop teaching affiliations for each of the municipal hospitals.

During his tenure as commissioner (1961–65), Dr. Trussel succeeded in developing contractual relationships for professional medical staff for all of the municipal hospitals except Sydenham, a small facility in Harlem to which community physicians admitted private patients, and Seaview, a chronic care hospital on Staten Island. The common element in the affiliation arrangements was payment of city funds on a cost-plus basis (direct costs plus an initial overhead rate of 10 percent) in exchange for provision of services by salaried physicians who would oversee the activities of municipal hospital interns and residents. In effect, all of the municipal hospitals (with the above-noted exceptions) became teaching hospitals, and the volunteer and part-time community physicians who had previously provided care were eliminated.

The more specific provisions of the affiliation contracts varied considerably, with ad hoc negotiations determining the outcomes. By 1965, 18 separate municipal facilities were affiliated with 17 different private institutions, including 5 of the city's 6 medical schools and 12 different voluntary teaching hospitals.[4] The range of services covered, the process for selection of house staff, and the degree of involvement of affiliates with hospital administration varied considerably. For example, only limited interdepartmental links were established between Columbia's College of Physicians and Surgeons and Harlem Hospital, while Montefiore Hospital assumed responsibility for all professional and auxiliary services at Morrisania Hospital, including nursing.

The affiliation contracts generally were successful in achieving their initial goal of improving the quality of physician services. Recruitment of staff at the municipal hospitals was greatly eased by the links with teaching institutions, although some of the hospitals that were affiliated with less well-known voluntary teaching hospitals were still obliged to depend heavily on foreign medical graduates. In addition, early critics pointed out that the close relations between public hospitals and voluntary teaching institutions could prove expensive, might sacrifice accountability in the management of public facilities, and could create pressures to underinvest in primary care while emphasizing tertiary care.[5]

## Table 3.1

### Medicaid Enrollments in New York City, 1968–84
### (in thousands)

| Year | Total | Public Assistance* | Medicaid Only |
|------|-------|--------------------|---------------|
| 1968 | 1,742.8 | 978.3 | 764.5 |
| 1969 | 1,903.8 | 1,039.3 | 864.5 |
| 1970 | 1,499.3 | 1,165.2 | 334.1 |
| 1971 | 1,618.2 | 1,251.1 | 367.1 |
| 1972 | 1,483.9 | 1,255.5 | 228.4 |
| 1973 | 1,363.3 | 1,170.1 | 193.2 |
| 1974 | 1,393.9 | 1,209.5 | 184.4 |
| 1975 | 1,421.0 | 1,266.2 | 154.8 |
| 1976 | 1,347.6 | 1,227.1 | 120.5 |
| 1977 | 1,272.9 | 1,171.8 | 101.1 |
| 1978 | 1,240.2 | 1,131.5 | 108.7 |
| 1979 | 1,189.9 | 1,099.6 | 90.3 |
| 1980 | 1,262.8 | 1,131.1 | 131.7 |
| 1981 | 1,161.2 | 1,034.7 | 126.5 |
| 1982 | 1,162.0 | 1,136.3 | 25.7 |
| 1983 | 1,194.1 | 1,167.0 | 27.1 |
| 1984 | 1,238.6 | 1,212.2 | 26.4 |

Sources: For 1968–78, data are from New York State Department of Social Services as reported in Charles Brecher and Diana Roswick, "The City's Role in Health Care," in Raymond D. Horton and Charles Brecher, eds., *Setting Municipal Priorities, 1980* (New York: Allenheld, Osmun and Co., 1979), p. 137; for 1979–84 the figures are from Office of Policy and Economic Research, *Dependency: An Economic and Social Data Report for New York City* (New York City Human Resources Administration, April 1985), Table 3.

*Includes SSI.

**Adjusting to Medicare and Medicaid.** Federal legislation in 1965 significantly changed the pattern of health care financing in the United States, with profound implications for New York City's municipal hospital system. The Medicare program provided direct federal funds to hospitals providing care to persons over age 65. The Medicaid program provided federal funds to aid states that created medical assistance programs for persons receiving public assistance and, at the states' option, for additional people with low incomes who did not qualify for cash assistance but were "medically needy." New York State responded quickly and in 1966 enacted a Medicaid program with a generous definition of medically needy. Enrollment grew rapidly to more than 1.9 million—about one-quarter of the city's population in 1969 (see Table 3.1). In addition, about 900,000 elderly New Yorkers qualified for Medicare. Given the widespread availability of group health insurance for the employed population, the expectation was that the new federal programs would ensure relatively good health coverage for virtually everyone in New York City.

The new federal and state programs were expected to be major sources of new funds for the municipal hospitals, which would both eliminate the historical underfunding by the city and permit service improvements. In fiscal year 1965, the budget for the Department of Hospitals was $242 million, over two-thirds of which was derived from local tax funds; by fiscal year 1971, the municipal hospitals were spending $663 million annually, with over one-half of the total coming from Medicare and Medicaid. These additional funds helped finance the growing affiliation program, permitted expansion of staff, and improved facilities.

Unfortunately, the fiscal boon from Medicaid and Medicare proved to be short-lived. The large Medicaid enrollments and the program's high costs caused it to be the first major social welfare program ever to be cut back by the state legislature. In 1969, income eligibility criteria were significantly reduced, causing enrollment to fall from 1.9 million to 1.5 million by 1970 (see Table 3.1). Subsequent near freezing of eligibility levels in the face of rapid inflation caused enrollment to continue to fall, to about 1.2 million New Yorkers in the early 1980s.

In the mid-1960s, with support from the federal Office of Economic Opportunity, the city health department launched a highly successful demonstration program to provide comprehensive ambulatory care services in a nontraditional clinic model at its Gouverneur health center.[6] With the availability of broad Medicaid coverage after 1967, Mayor John V. Lindsay decided to expand this approach to virtually all of the city's ambulatory care operations. As part of a broader reorganization of city government, the health and hospitals departments were merged into a single health services administration, the head of the Gouverneur clinic was made head of the new agency, and planning was launched for a citywide network of neighborhood family care centers (NFCCs). The plan called initially for 31 centers, located in all boroughs, with an estimated capital cost of $100 million. Some of the facilities would be at older municipal hospitals whose inpatient services were scheduled for closure or replacement, but most were to be in new buildings. The combination of higher-than-expected costs for the NFCCs and the sharp cutbacks in Medicaid eligibility led city budget officials to argue successfully for reductions in the NFCC program. The notion of separate facilities providing conveniently located, family-oriented ambulatory care remained a goal of the municipal hospitals, but implementation of the NFCC model was limited to a few sites.

The availability of Medicaid and Medicare funds also led city officials to accelerate and expand plans for construction of new municipal hospital facilities. Major capital projects were authorized in several hospitals. Since the new facilities replaced ward arrangements with semiprivate rooms (to meet Medicaid and Medicare standards) and included more sophisticated equipment, they also generally required increased operating costs compared to the costs of the facilities they replaced. In the case of Woodhull Hospital, the desire to avoid the higher operating costs led city officials to delay fully opening the facility until the early 1980s.

In addition to their financing implications, Medicare and Medicaid also had serious long-run effects on the demand for health care by the elderly and indigent and on the share of that demand that the municipal hospitals were required to meet. In the years following enactment of the federal programs, the number of general care hospital discharges from all facilities in the city rose from slightly over 1,000,000 in 1967 to an all-time high of 1,154,000 in 1972 (see Table 3.2).

The new program enabled members of the Medicare population to have greater choice in their source of hospitalization. In the early 1960s, the municipal hospitals cared for about one-third of all hospitalized persons over age 65; by 1970, the municipal share had fallen to under 18 percent, and by 1975 to under 13 percent.[7]

For the nonaged indigent, the initial effect of Medicaid also was to eliminate the financial barrier to care at voluntary hospitals, but access remained limited because these people often did not have relationships with the private physicians who generated the bulk of voluntary hospital admissions. Thus, the initial shifts from municipal to voluntary hospitals were less dramatic for the Medicaid population than for the Medicare population, but the program nonetheless reduced demand for municipal inpatient services. General care discharges from municipal hospitals numbered 218,000, or 21 percent of the citywide total in 1965; the figure fell immediately following passage of the new programs but rose again following the state's Medicaid eligibility cutbacks. During the remainder of the 1970s, an industrywide trend toward fewer admissions reduced the citywide total, but declines in the Medicaid-enrolled population helped stabilize the municipal hospitals' share (see Table 3.2). That is, the limits on Medicaid eligibility since the early 1970s have reduced the number and share of the indigent population enrolled in the program, and those indigent not covered by Medicaid have been obliged to rely heavily on the municipal system.

The Medicaid program had fiscal implications that extended

## Table 3.2

## General Care Discharges in New York City, 1965–84
### (numbers in thousands)

| | *Voluntary* | | *Municipal* | | *Proprietary* | | *State* | | *Total Discharges per Year* | |
|---|---|---|---|---|---|---|---|---|---|---|
| *Year* | *No.* | *%* | *No.* | *%* | *No.* | *%* | *No.* | *%* | *No.* | *%* |
| 1965 | 669 | 64.1 | 218 | 20.9 | 156 | 15.0 | 0 | 0.0 | 1,043 | 100.0 |
| 1966 | 663 | 64.5 | 211 | 20.5 | 154 | 15.0 | 0 | 0.0 | 1,028 | 100.0 |
| 1967 | 648 | 64.5 | 200 | 12.0 | 153 | 15.2 | 3 | 0.3 | 1,004 | 100.0 |
| 1968 | 652 | 64.6 | 198 | 19.6 | 153 | 15.2 | 5 | 0.5 | 1,008 | 100.0 |
| 1969 | 657 | 65.4 | 190 | 18.9 | 151 | 15.0 | 6 | 0.6 | 1,004 | 100.0 |
| 1970 | 698 | 64.3 | 211 | 19.4 | 172 | 15.9 | 7 | 0.6 | 1,088 | 100.0 |
| 1971 | 718 | 62.3 | 228 | 19.8 | 200 | 17.4 | 7 | 0.6 | 1,153 | 100.0 |
| 1972 | 732 | 63.4 | 218 | 18.9 | 196 | 17.0 | 9 | 0.8 | 1,155 | 100.0 |
| 1973 | 729 | 64.9 | 214 | 19.1 | 171 | 15.2 | 8 | 0.7 | 1,122 | 100.0 |
| 1974 | 743 | 66.3 | 212 | 18.9 | 158 | 14.1 | 9 | 0.8 | 1,122 | 100.0 |
| 1975 | 761 | 67.6 | 204 | 18.1 | 152 | 13.5 | 10 | 0.9 | 1,127 | 100.0 |
| 1976 | 764 | 69.9 | 187 | 17.1 | 133 | 12.2 | 9 | 0.8 | 1,093 | 100.0 |
| 1977 | 773 | 70.5 | 198 | 18.0 | 117 | 10.7 | 9 | 0.8 | 1,097 | 100.0 |
| 1978 | 762 | 70.7 | 213 | 19.8 | 92 | 8.5 | 10 | 0.9 | 1,077 | 100.0 |
| 1979 | 770 | 70.6 | 216 | 19.8 | 93 | 8.5 | 12 | 1.1 | 1,091 | 100.0 |
| 1980 | 798 | 72.2 | 210 | 19.0 | 84 | 7.6 | 12 | 1.1 | 1,104 | 100.0 |
| 1981 | 801 | 72.2 | 212 | 19.1 | 84 | 7.6 | 12 | 1.1 | 1,109 | 100.0 |
| 1982 | 815 | 72.2 | 218 | 19.3 | 85 | 7.5 | 11 | 1.0 | 1,129 | 100.0 |
| 1983 | 813 | 72.1 | 219 | 19.4 | 85 | 7.5 | 11 | 1.0 | 1,128 | 100.0 |
| 1984 | 814 | 71.8 | 226 | 19.9 | 82 | 7.2 | 11 | 1.0 | 1,133 | 100.0 |

*Source: Profiles and Trends, Hospital Inpatient and Ambulatory Care in Southern New York* (New York: United Hospital Fund, 1986).

beyond the financing of the municipal hospital system. When the state created the program, it followed the model established for public assistance programs and required localities to share equally the costs of the program not federally reimbursed. Given the federal cost-sharing formulas and the existence of a component of the program that is not federally reimbursed, the city's share of total Medicaid expenditures has been about 29 percent.

The city has had to provide local tax funds for its share of costs for medical services to the indigent outside of municipal hospitals. These costs have far outgrown the amounts the city paid prior to Medicaid to voluntary hospitals for medical services for the poor. In 1965, the city spent about $102 million for purchases of private (i.e., nonmunicipal hospital) medical care for the indigent, with most of the funds coming from local sources. By 1970, the total cost of private services under Medicaid was over $454 million and the city's share of $136 million more than exceeded its pre-Medicaid commitment.[8] This fiscal obligation has grown steadily since 1970. The city's share of Medicaid payments for purchases from the private sector exceeded $300 million by 1975 and was estimated at $800 million in 1985.

The city's dual role as partial financier of a state-controlled program of medical purchases and as sponsor of a large hospital system places it in a difficult position with regard to statewide Medicaid policy. In its role as financier, the city endorses measures for cost control and limitations on total expenditures; but in its role as the sponsor of the municipal hospitals, the city seeks maximum Medicaid payments because the local subsidy is derived entirely from local tax funds. Thus, the city is constantly evaluating Medicaid policy in terms of increased revenues for municipal hospitals versus the additional municipal expenditures for other providers. Except for continuing to call for a reduced local share in the total financing, the city has been relatively cautious in its pursuit of changes in the Medicaid program. The city's pleas for a lower share of Medicaid costs were largely ignored in the state legislature until the early 1980s, when a reduction in the required city share for selected long-term care services was enacted.

**The Creation of the Health and Hospitals Corporation.** The enactment of federal Medicaid and Medicare legislation in 1965 coincided with the election of a reform mayor in New York City. The new mayor, John V. Lindsay, had promised improved municipal hospitals as part of his campaign. The new federal programs made this goal appear realistic. Lindsay appointed a blue-ribbon commission under the chairmanship of Gerard Piel in 1966. In 1967 the commission reported with a call for fundamental changes in the local health care system.

The Piel Commission's goal was elimination of the dual system of health care that had lower standards for the poor. The members believed that Medicare and Medicaid not only would provide the resources to accomplish this goal but also justified a stronger public role in managing the entire city's health care system. Under Medicare and Medicaid the voluntary hospitals were likely to be deriving more than one-half of their revenues from public sources, which in the minds of commission members justified public control over all health care institutions in the city. The commission was also concerned about the operation of the municipal hospitals and sought to improve the management of the hospitals by reducing the degree to which they were overseen by the citywide budget and personnel agencies.

The commission recommended creation of a new public benefit corporation, the Health Services Corporation, that would be responsible for coordinating all public funds for health care in the city and be able to use this leverage to establish regional networks of facilities consisting of both municipal and voluntary institutions. It would collect third-party revenues but also receive a lump-sum payment from the city. The new corporation also would be responsible for operating the municipal hospitals without the constraints of a civil service system or reliance on centralized municipal purchasing agencies. The corporation would be governed by a board of nine prominent citizens, none of whom would be employees of the city, to be appointed by the mayor.

In 1969, a political agreement was forged among the mayor, the city council, and the municipal hospitals employees' union leaders that resulted in state legislation creating the New York City Health and Hospitals Corporation (HHC). The HHC was given responsibility for operating the municipal hospitals and other health care facilities that the city might assign it. Ownership of the facilities as well as responsibility for capital improvements remained with the city. However, the HHC was responsible for collecting all third-party revenues and would be given a lump-sum appropriation from the city. The amount of the city subsidy was set at $175 million in the first year, with subsequent adjustments for inflation and changes in the responsibilities the city asked the HHC to undertake. The HHC was freed from direct control by the city's budget agency and was able to make its own purchasing arrangements. In addition, the HHC was empowered to create subsidiary corporations to operate individual facilities, a provision included to permit greater decentralization of municipal hospital operations.

While the HHC incorporated some of the structural features recommended by the Piel Commission, the compromises necessary to obtain the authorizing legislation led to several important deviations from the original model. The HHC's board was expanded to 16 people, with more responsiveness to the local political establishment than the commission recommended. To gain the support of the union leaders, the legislation provided civil service protection for all nonmanagerial municipal hospital employees and retained the municipal employees' union as collective bargaining agent; also, informal commitments were made to the union to limit and eventually reduce the hiring of nonphysician personnel through the affiliation contracts.

The HHC began operations on 1 July 1970, with little lead time for planning. In its early years it continued to rely heavily on the city overhead agencies for personnel, purchasing, and financial management. Since it inherited a weak billing and collections system from the Department of Hospitals, the HHC found it could not achieve initial targets for third-party revenue collections and thus was obliged to rely on the city for working capital. Financial autonomy and greater management flexibility proved difficult to achieve. Because of its numerous early difficulties the HHC was viewed by many as a disappointment. In 1973, a state study commission issued a well-publicized report concluding that "the people of New York City are not being materially better served by the Health and Hospitals Corporation than by its predecessor agencies."[9]

Despite its poor image, the HHC accomplished three important things during its first five years. First, improved billing and accounting systems caused collections from third parties to increase significantly. In the last year of operations by the Department of Hospitals, about one-half of the $522 million budget was covered through third-party collections.[10] In its first year the HHC collected about 65 percent of its budget from third parties, and the amounts rose steadily to approximately 70 percent in the mid-1970s (see Table 3.3).

Second, during the early years the HHC board attained some independence politically and took on the role of health care advocate. Mayor Lindsay appointed to the board several prominent citizens who pursued expansion of the HHC's programs. In 1972, the board even sued the city to force it to increase its annual payments.

Third, the HHC expanded its outpatient services significantly in the early 1970s. The HHC assumed responsibility for some ambulatory care services formerly under the Department of Health and expanded its own efforts. From 1971 to 1975, the number of outpatient visits to HHC facilities grew from 3.1 million to 5.0 million. The later year's total includes numerous nonphysician visits, often to methadone maintenance clinics previously operated by the health department.

**Effects of the 1975 Fiscal Crisis.** In early 1975, the city of New York was revealed to have sizable budget deficits and was denied access to public credit markets. As a result, the city was obliged by its creditors to make substantial cuts in its expenditures, including layoffs of municipal employees. The city also was placed under the supervision of an emergency financial control board (later the financial control board, or FCB) dominated by the governor. Also placed under the scrutiny of the FCB were several semiautonomous or "covered" agencies dependent on city funds, including the HHC.

The immediate effect of the fiscal crisis was sharp staff reductions and severe expenditure limits for the HHC. The HHC payroll (excluding affiliate employees) had grown from 40,036 in 1971 to 49,080 in 1975; in the next three years it was cut 17 percent to 41,892 and then reached a low of 40,431 in 1980 (see Table 3.4). Total HHC expenditures, which had risen 54 percent—from $663 million to

$1,021 million between 1970 and 1975—were virtually frozen for the next five years and reached only $1,170 million in 1980 (see Table 3.3).

The volume of inpatient services provided by the HHC was affected only modestly by these resource reductions. However, a trend toward reduced lengths of stay meant that the HHC's continued provision of care to the same number of people admitted required fewer days of care and hence fewer hospital beds. The HHC had almost an identical number of general care admissions in 1972 and 1982, but the average length of stay fell from 11 days to 8.3 days. Accordingly, the number of days of care fell almost 23 percent during this period.

The reductions in lengths of stay and total days of care were accompanied by reductions in the bed capacity of the HHC system (see Table 3.5). Between 1975 and 1980, inpatient general care services were closed at Morrisania, Gouverneur, Francis Delafield, Fordham, and Sydenham hospitals, and the bed capacity of most other HHC facilities was reduced. For example, Metropolitan Hospital, which was at one time targeted for closure but remained open, saw its general care bed capacity cut from 626 beds in 1975 to 522 beds in 1980 and 407 beds in 1984. For all HHC hospitals, the decline in general care bed capacity was 16 percent between 1975 and 1980.

The fiscal crisis also helped bring about changes in the relationships between the HHC and the city general government. As noted above, the fiscal monitors established by the state exercised supervision over the HHC as well as the city. The procedures developed for financial planning delegated responsibility to the city for submitting a plan for the HHC that was consistent with the city's own budget. That is, the HHC had to develop a budget that required no more city funds than the city was including in its financial plan for the HHC, and this figure had to be viewed as reasonable by the fiscal monitors. The effect of this coordinated financial oversight was to give the city more direct control over HHC budget planning and to make the processes of both agencies subject to greater public scrutiny. After some initial battles between the HHC leadership and the FCB, which eventually led to the dismissal of an HHC president in 1976, the city's Office of Management and Budget (OMB) and the HHC developed smoother working relationships for arriving at compatible financial plans.

The need to contain spending and the desire to reduce HHC bed capacity also led Mayor Edward I. Koch, who took office in 1978, to seek greater political control over the HHC board and to involve his appointees more closely in the management of the HHC. During

## Table 3.3

## Financing of the HHC, Fiscal Years 1971–77
### (dollars in millions)

| | 1971 $ | 1971 % | 1972 $ | 1972 % | 1973 $ | 1973 % | 1974 $ | 1974 % | 1975 $ | 1975 % | 1976 $ | 1976 % | 1977 $ | 1977 % |
|---|---|---|---|---|---|---|---|---|---|---|---|---|---|---|
| **Revenues** | | | | | | | | | | | | | | |
| Third-party | | | | | | | | | | | | | | |
| Medicaid | 296 | 44.6 | 322 | 46.7 | 436 | 54.8 | 436 | 50.3 | 467 | 45.7 | 495 | 46.8 | 406 | 40.0 |
| Medicare | 50 | 7.5 | 53 | 7.7 | 43 | 5.4 | 77 | 8.9 | 110 | 10.8 | 136 | 12.9 | 131 | 12.9 |
| Blue Cross[a] | 86 | 13.0 | 73 | 10.6 | 96 | 12.1 | 115 | 13.3 | 113 | 11.1 | 132 | 12.5 | 40 | 3.9 |
| Other[a] | – | – | – | – | – | – | – | – | – | – | – | – | 43 | 4.2 |
| Subtotal | 432 | 65.2 | 448 | 64.9 | 575 | 72.2 | 628 | 72.5 | 690 | 67.6 | 763 | 72.2 | 620 | 61.0 |
| N.Y.C. subsidy | 231 | 34.8 | 242 | 35.1 | 221 | 27.8 | 238 | 27.5 | 331 | 32.4 | 294 | 27.8 | 365[b] | 36.0 |
| Other | 0 | – | 0 | – | 0 | – | 0 | – | 0 | – | 0 | – | 30 | 3.0 |
| Total | 663 | 100.0 | 690 | 100.0 | 796 | 100.0 | 866 | 100.0 | 1,021 | 100.0 | 1,057 | 100.0 | 1,015 | 100.0 |
| **Expenditures** | | | | | | | | | | | | | | |
| Affiliation contracts | NA[c] | – | NA | – | NA | – | NA | – | NA | – | NA | – | 149 | 14.7 |
| Other | NA | – | NA | – | NA | – | NA | – | NA | – | NA | – | 865 | 85.3 |
| Total | 663 | 100.0 | 690 | 100.0 | 796 | 100.0 | 866 | 100.0 | 1,021 | 100.0 | 1,058 | 100.0 | 1,014 | 100.0 |

Sources: Figures for FYs 1971–76 are budget figures reported in Charles Brecher and Diana Roswick, "The City's Role in Health Care," in Raymond D. Horton and Charles Brecher, eds., *Setting Municipal Priorities, 1980* (New York: Allenheld, Osmun and Co., 1979), p. 156; figures for FY 1977 are calculated from *New York City Health and Hospitals Corporation Financial Statements for Years Ended 1977 and 1978* (New York: Arthur Andersen & Company, 1979).

[a]For FYs 1971–76, figures shown are for revenues from Blue Cross and other payers combined. Separate figures were not available for these years.

[b]Subsidy figure includes change in fund balance for the Health and Hospitals Corporation. The city tax levy appropriation was $324 million in FY 1977.

[c]NA: Not available.

*Continued*

## Table 3.3—Continued
## Fiscal Years 1978–86
### (dollars in millions)

| | 1978 $ | 1978 % | 1979 $ | 1979 % | 1980 $ | 1980 % | 1981 $ | 1981 % | 1982 $ | 1982 % | 1983 $ | 1983 % | 1984 $ | 1984 % | 1985 $ | 1985 % | 1986 $ | 1986 % |
|---|---|---|---|---|---|---|---|---|---|---|---|---|---|---|---|---|---|---|
| **Revenues** | | | | | | | | | | | | | | | | | | |
| Third-party | | | | | | | | | | | | | | | | | | |
| Medicaid | 389 | 35.4 | 379 | 35.2 | 397 | 33.9 | 506 | 38.0 | 661 | 45.0 | 740 | 46.2 | 849 | 47.6 | 913 | 46.0 | 969[e] | 46.9 |
| Medicare | 143 | 13.0 | 177 | 16.4 | 209 | 17.9 | 260 | 19.5 | 275 | 18.7 | 282 | 17.6 | 295 | 16.5 | 275 | 13.9 | 277[e] | 13.4 |
| Blue Cross | 42 | 3.8 | 42 | 3.9 | 51 | 4.4 | 60 | 4.5 | 89 | 6.1 | 93 | 5.8 | 94 | 5.3 | 92 | 4.6 | 99 | 4.8 |
| Other | 60 | 5.5 | 53 | 4.9 | 61 | 5.2 | 65 | 4.9 | 75 | 5.1 | 84 | 5.2 | 90 | 5.0 | 105 | 5.3 | 127 | 5.9 |
| Subtotal | 634 | 57.6 | 651 | 60.4 | 718 | 61.4 | 891 | 66.9 | 1,100 | 74.8 | 1,199 | 74.9 | 1,328 | 74.4 | 1,385 | 69.9 | 1,472 | 71.0 |
| N.Y.C. subsidy | 427[d] | 38.9 | 404 | 37.5 | 429 | 36.7 | 416 | 31.3 | 348 | 23.7 | 386 | 24.1 | 419 | 23.5 | 597 | 30.1 | 598 | 29.0 |
| Other | 39 | 3.5 | 22 | 2.0 | 23 | 2.0 | 24 | 1.8 | 22 | 1.5 | 16 | 1.0 | 38 | 2.1 | 0 | – | 0 | – |
| Total | 1,100 | 100.0 | 1,077 | 100.0 | 1,170 | 100.0 | 1,331 | 100.0 | 1,470 | 100.0 | 1,601 | 100.0 | 1,785 | 100.0 | 1,982 | 100.0 | 2,070 | 100.0 |
| **Expenditures** | | | | | | | | | | | | | | | | | | |
| Affiliation contracts | 156 | 14.2 | 168 | 16.0 | 179 | 15.3 | 199 | 15.2 | 217 | 14.8 | 232 | 14.5 | 262 | 14.7 | 270 | 14.7 | 284 | 13.8 |
| Other | 943 | 85.8 | 883 | 84.0 | 991 | 84.7 | 1,114 | 84.8 | 1,253 | 85.2 | 1,369 | 85.5 | 1,523 | 85.3 | 1,712 | 85.3 | 1,786 | 86.2 |
| Total | 1,099 | 100.0 | 1,051 | 100.0 | 1,170 | 100.0 | 1,313 | 100.0 | 1,470 | 100.0 | 1,601 | 100.0 | 1,785 | 100.0 | 1,982 | 100.0 | 2,070 | 100.0 |

Sources: Figures for FY 1978 are calculated from *New York City Health and Hospitals Corporation Financial Statements for Years Ended 1978 and 1979* (New York: Arthur Andersen & Company, 1980). For FYs 1979–84, figures are from New York City Health and Hospitals Corporation, "Finance Briefing Memo," December 1984. Figures for FY 1985 provided by City of New York, Office of Management and Budget. Figures for FY 1986 are from New York State Financial Control Board, "Staff Report on Modification No. 86–13 to New York City's FYs 1986–1989 Financial Plan," February 1986.

[d]Subsidy figure includes change in fund balance for the Health and Hospitals Corporation. The city tax levy appropriation was $362 million for FY 1978.

[e]Net of disallowances.

**Table 3.4**

**HHC Staff, Fiscal Years 1971–85**

| | 1971 | 1975 | 1978 | 1979 | 1980 | 1981 | 1982 | 1983 | 1984 | 1985 |
|---|---|---|---|---|---|---|---|---|---|---|
| HHC corporate staff | 40,036 | 49,080 | 41,892 | 40,683 | 40,431 | 41,317 | 41,628 | 42,220 | 43,751 | 43,568 |
| Affiliated staff | NA | NA | 4,793 | 4,699 | 4,848 | 4,848* | 4,682 | 4,656 | 5,359 | 5,378 |
| Full-time-equivalent physicians | NA | NA | 2,082 | 2,021 | 2,213 | 2,213 | 1,292 | 1,511 | 1,968 | 1,951 |
| Full-time-equivalent nonphysicians | NA | NA | 2,711 | 2,678 | 2,635 | 2,635 | 3,390 | 3,145 | 3,391 | 3,427 |
| Total | NA | NA | 46,685 | 45,382 | 45,279 | 46,165 | 46,310 | 46,876 | 49,110 | 48,946 |

Sources: For 1978–85, "Mayor's Management Report" (New York City Office of Operations, 20 August 1979 and supplements 17 September 1980, 17 September 1982, 30 January 1984, and 14 February 1985; for earlier years, James Hartman, "Expenditures and Services," in Raymond D. Horton and Charles Brecher, eds., *Setting Municipal Priorities, 1980* (New York: Allenheld, Osmun and Co., 1979), Table 3.6.

*Actual figures are not available. Data shown are those planned for FY 1981.

NA: Not available.

Mayor Koch's first term this goal led to conflict with three successive HHC presidents (Joseph Lynaugh, Joseph Hoffman, and Abraham Kauvar), each of whom served only a relatively short period before leaving over disagreements with the mayor. In 1981, Mayor Koch selected, and the board approved, Stanley Brezenoff as president. Brezenoff had served as a commissioner since 1978 and brought to the office of president both organizational stability and personal loyalty to the mayor. Brezenoff was elevated to deputy mayor in 1984, but he recruited his successors in the HHC and they served under him. The combination of new board appointees by Mayor Koch and selection of presidents sensitive to the mayor's desire to exercise close control over HHC have changed HHC's character. Instead of being a semiautonomous body, it operates much like other mayoral agencies.

**Recent Initiatives.** In 1981, the city achieved a balanced budget; the local fiscal climate has improved since. In 1982 Mayor Koch successfully ran for reelection with promises to expand and improve services; since then new resources have been devoted to the HHC. In addition, a new state program for hospital reimbursement by Medicaid, Medicare, and Blue Cross, adopted in 1982, has provided additional resources through both increased reimbursement rates and special earmarked funds for care for the medically indigent. Moreover, the more stable management of the HHC in the early 1980s facilitated realization of many of the collections improvements planned in earlier years.

As a result of this combination of circumstances, the HHC budget was increased more than 50 percent, from $1,170 million in 1980 to $1,785 million in 1984. The share of revenues derived from third parties increased from 61 percent in 1980 to nearly 75 percent in 1984 (see Table 3.3). Thus, the HHC financed most of its budgetary expansion through third-party revenues rather than city subsidies.

The new revenues, together with a more harmonious relationship with city officials, have enabled the HHC to undertake several pro-grammatic initiatives in recent years. Six of these efforts are described briefly below.[11]

The HHC acute care hospitals have suffered from a chronic shortage of nursing personnel, particularly registered nurses. Since 1981, increased funding expanded the number of registered nurses 29 percent, from 5,098 in 1981 to 6,565 in 1985. However, HHC still has to rely on per diem nurses to meet a substantial portion of its needs. Accordingly, programs have been launched to enhance recruiting and to reduce expenses for per diem nurses, including a flexible work schedule program, forgivable loans for senior nursing students, and a

## Table 3.5

### HHC General Care Bed Complement, 1965–74

| Hospital | 1965 | 1966 | 1967 | 1968 | 1969 | 1970 | 1971 | 1972 | 1973 | 1974 |
|---|---|---|---|---|---|---|---|---|---|---|
| Bronx Municipal | 858 | 793 | 802 | 793 | 767 | 781 | 786 | 780 | 775 | 740 |
| Fordham | 414 | 416 | 416 | 416 | 401 | 401 | 406 | 406 | 406 | 406 |
| Lincoln | 359 | 345 | 354 | 354 | 350 | 350 | 350 | 346 | 343 | 302 |
| Morrisania | 402 | 402 | 366 | 366 | 331 | 331 | 331 | 309 | 313 | 307 |
| Coney Island | 495 | 421 | 395 | 404 | 404 | 408 | 408 | 408 | 382 | 420 |
| Cumberland | 378 | 303 | 354 | 348 | 371 | 359 | 366 | 368 | 368 | 346 |
| Greenpoint | 205 | 178 | 177 | 177 | 174 | 174 | 174 | 174 | 174 | 174 |
| Kings County Hospital Center | 1,683 | 1,668 | 1,668 | 1,616 | 1,551 | 1,585 | 1,577 | 1,504 | 1,365 | 1,157 |
| Bellevue | 1,685 | 1,523 | 1,456 | 1,489 | 1,142 | 1,142 | 1,131 | 1,140 | 1,014 | 955 |
| Francis Delafield | 295 | 259 | 255 | 255 | 261 | 261 | 250 | 250 | 250 | 231 |
| Harlem | 825 | 781 | 777 | 777 | 755 | 809 | 809 | 799 | 801 | 797 |
| James Ewing | 263 | 240 | 240 | 240 | C | C | C | C | C | C |
| Metropolitan | 794 | 774 | 766 | 758 | 723 | 723 | 726 | 735 | 735 | 659 |
| Sydenham | 218 | 218 | 218 | 216 | 216 | 209 | 209 | 207 | 173 | 196 |
| City Hospital at Elmhurst | 636 | 619 | 619 | 613 | 651 | 651 | 651 | 659 | 653 | 662 |
| Queens Hospital Center | 783 | 854 | 781 | 866 | 855 | 874 | 874 | 880 | 878 | 701 |
| Gouverneur | C | C | C | C | C | C | C | C | 71 | 119 |
| North Central Bronx | | | | | | | | | | |
| Woodhull | | | | | | | | | | |
| Total | 10,293 | 9,794 | 9,644 | 9,688 | 8,952 | 9,058 | 9,048 | 8,965 | 8,701 | 8,172 |

Sources: Health and Hospital Planning Council of Southern New York, "Hospitals and Related Facilities in Southern New York," 1965–75 editions. United Hospital Fund, "Hospitals and Related Facilities in Southern New York," 1976–84 editions. Data for 1984 provided by the United Hospital Fund.

C: Closed.

Continued

# Table 3.5—Continued
## HHC General Care Bed Complement, 1975-84

| Hospital | 1975 | 1976 | 1977 | 1978 | 1979 | 1980 | 1981 | 1982* | 1983* | 1984* |
|---|---|---|---|---|---|---|---|---|---|---|
| Bronx Municipal | 724 | 717 | 720 | 690 | 658 | 656 | 642 | 640 | 640 | 640 |
| Fordham | 406 | 387 | C | C | C | C | C | C | C | C |
| Lincoln | 292 | 292 | 383 | 509 | 509 | 509 | 509 | 513 | 517 | 517 |
| Morrisania | 311 | 303 | C | C | C | C | C | C | C | C |
| Coney Island | 408 | 387 | 378 | 378 | 378 | 378 | 374 | 374 | 374 | 374 |
| Cumberland | 334 | 334 | 334 | 310 | 310 | 310 | 264 | 257 | C | C |
| Greenpoint | 174 | 174 | 174 | 174 | 174 | 174 | 156 | C | C | C |
| Kings County Hospital Center | 1,138 | 1,110 | 1,089 | 1,038 | 1,021 | 1,008 | 878 | 878 | 877 | 877 |
| Bellevue | 828 | 793 | 847 | 862 | 858 | 789 | 789 | 786 | 786 | 786 |
| Francis Delafield | 195 | C | C | C | C | C | C | C | C | C |
| Harlem | 793 | 799 | 770 | 770 | 688 | 688 | 667 | 658 | 639 | 639 |
| James Ewing | C | C | C | C | C | C | C | C | C | C |
| Metropolitan | 626 | 619 | 588 | 566 | 576 | 522 | 460 | 450 | 407 | 407 |
| Sydenham | 193 | 169 | 129 | 132 | 132 | 120 | C | C | C | C |
| City Hospital at Elmhurst | 654 | 587 | 621 | 593 | 583 | 583 | 521 | 509 | 493 | 493 |
| Queens Hospital Center | 673 | 623 | 618 | 600 | 540 | 540 | 460 | 455 | 458 | 454 |
| Gouveneur | 119 | 104 | 0 | C | C | C | C | C | C | C |
| North Central Bronx | | | 157 | 306 | 347 | 352 | 352 | 350 | 341 | 347 |
| Woodhull | | | | | | | | 94 | 238 | 322 |
| Total | 7,868 | 7,398 | 6,808 | 6,928 | 6,774 | 6,629 | 6,072 | 5,964 | 5,770 | 5,856 |

*Certified beds; bed complement not published.
C: Closed.

career ladder program for practical nurses. In 1983, the HHC created a subsidiary corporation, Nurse Registry, Inc., to provide per diem nurses and make it possible to reduce overtime. This agency provides nurses to nine municipal hospitals.

Another chronic problem for HHC hospitals has been poorly equipped and poorly staffed medical records units. In recognition of the need for better medical records, the HHC launched a "medical records initiative" in 1982 that provided additional funds as well as central office management attention to deal with the problem. Over the next three years the initiative reduced the number of incomplete records at most facilities. By 1985, all hospitals except Kings County met the state standard of having at least 50 percent of all records up to date within 15 days of a patient's discharge.

In March of 1982, the HHC created a task force to develop improved standards for the affiliation contracts — another of the HHC's continuing concerns. In subsequent years more detailed contracts replaced commonplace letters of intent, specifying minimum standards for coverage of obstetrics, anesthesia, radiology, and emergency room services; they also transferred responsibility for some support services from the affiliate to the HHC. In addition, a new central office unit was created to negotiate and monitor the contracts.

A major effort of the HHC board and staff in recent years has been to serve better its role as family doctor to most of the city's poorer residents. In November of 1982, the board adopted a formal ambulatory care initiative, which called for the reorganization of most high-volume clinics into family-oriented services staffed by primary care teams. By mid-1985 this program had been implemented in the general medicine and pediatric clinics of 10 acute care hospitals, the obstetric and gynecological services of 4 hospitals, and five of the six NFCCs in all three services.

A state policy to reduce the number of mentally ill persons cared for at the state's mental hospitals has created chronic overcrowding in municipal psychiatric acute care units. The HHC has sought to address this problem by better coordinating patient admission to state facilities, by enlarging HHC psychiatric facilities, and by expanding HHC outpatient mental health services. In addition, new psychiatric ambulatory care programs were launched, including one aimed at homeless individuals.

The city of New York's achievement of a balanced budget in the early 1980s and its subsequent return to public credit markets permitted the city to develop a long-run capital program for its hospitals. In cooperation with the city's OMB, the HHC prepared its first 10-year capital plan in 1983. The capital plan provides for expenditures of over $1.5 billion during the next decade. Nearly two-thirds of the funds are allocated for major reconstruction of five hospitals. Two of the hospitals (Kings County and Queens) are among the oldest HHC facilities; the other three (Elmhurst, Coney Island, and Bronx Municipal) were built in the 1950s. The remainder of the funds is for equipment and routine rehabilitation or reconstruction. Specification of the reconstruction requirements for the new facilities is a major current effort of the HHC planning staff.

The foregoing six efforts represent initiatives aimed at most of the major concerns of HHC top management during the 1981–85 period. More recently, new challenges have emerged, including the need to treat growing numbers of patients with acquired immune deficiency syndrome and the changes in federal and state reimbursement policy that followed expiration of the federal waiver at the end of 1985. The changes in the reimbursement policy, which shifted payment from a per diem to a per-case basis for Medicare in 1986 and for other payers in 1988, could slow or even reverse HHC's recent financial gains.

**Regulatory Climate.** The HHC operates its facilities in a health care market that is perhaps the most heavily regulated in the nation. The principal regulatory tools have been twofold: certificate of need (CON) requirements that oblige hospitals to demonstrate a societal need for capital investments before the capital investments can be made, and the setting of rates at which third parties can pay hospitals for their services.

These regulatory tools have been used to reduce the supply of hospital beds statewide and in New York City and to reduce the rate of increase in operating expenditures. In addition, the state has proposed to extend its regulatory authority to reduce graduate medical education programs in the state and to promote more training for primary care specialties. Related state initiatives are proposed changes in rate-setting policy that would shift payment for capital expenses and graduate medical education from a historical base to statewide pools to be distributed according to policies established by the state health commissioner.

*Certificate of need.* New York, with its 1964 legislation, was the first state to enact CON controls over hospital construction. Other states later adopted similar approaches, and federal health planning legislation mandated CON programs for all states in 1974. More recently, the Reagan administration and Congress have eased federal requirements, but New York has continued its strong controls over capital programs.

Initially, the state delegated project review authority for the New

York City area to a local health and hospitals planning council that was dominated by providers, specifically by the large voluntary hospitals. This body favored expansion of large voluntary institutions and closure of smaller institutions — policies generally consistent with municipal plans to rebuild selected institutions, generally on a smaller scale, and to reconfigure facilities for better affiliation arrangements with the large teaching institutions. A notable example was the construction of North Central Bronx Hospital, adjacent to its affiliate, Montefiore Hospital, as a replacement for two closed hospitals located in the South Bronx.

In the early 1970s, the provider-dominated planning agency was replaced, in accordance with federal guidelines, with local and state planning bodies containing more consumer representation but ultimately accountable to the governor. For most of the 1970s, capital investment regulation was not a significant issue for the HHC. Most of its construction efforts were completion of renovations approved in the earlier decade. This resulted in the previously noted 27 percent reduction in bed supply during the 1970s, consistent with state and planning agency goals.

With the availability of new capital resources in the 1980s and the development of a 10-year capital plan, the HHC envisages rebuilding five hospitals, though specific plans indicating their bed size and service mix have not yet been formulated. In all likelihood, state officials will use their CON authority to question, if not limit, the size and character of the facilities the HHC anticipates building over the next decade.

*Rate regulation.* State rate setting has been a pressing concern for the HHC in recent years and may be a troublesome issue in the future. The state legislature permitted prospective controls on hospital payments in 1970 in response to rapidly increasing Blue Cross premiums and escalating Medicaid expenditures, but it was not until the city's and state's fiscal problems in the mid-1970s that rate-setting authority was used aggressively to slow increases in hospital revenues. Caps were placed on Medicaid outpatient payments, and controls were devised for inpatient per diem costs. These policies seriously affected HHC revenues because of the HHC's large outpatient work load and its large share of Medicaid patients at the same time that the city's subsidy was squeezed by its fiscal crisis. These circumstances help explain the almost stable HHC budget during the 1975–80 period (see Table 3.3).

The limitations on third-party revenues also had serious consequences for many voluntary hospitals. Because they were not able to control expenditures adequately, many such institutions dipped into reserves to cover operating costs. Virtually all voluntary hospitals in New York City had operating deficits; many were concerned about their viability under continued state rate-setting policies.

In response, the state developed a new reimbursement policy in 1982, known as the New York prospective hospital reimbursement methodology, or NYPHRM. It maintained prospective limits on per diem payments and extended the scope of regulation to commercial payers and Medicare. This extended regulation of "all payers" was accepted by the hospitals in exchange for additional revenues, to be paid out of a newly created pool of funds, to cover the costs of bad debt and charity care. The new pool of money was created by payments from third parties, including the state and federal governments. The federal government granted the state a three-year Medicare waiver to experiment with the new system.

In creating the new system, the state was primarily concerned with the voluntary institutions, less so with the public hospitals. In fact, the state and the voluntary sector wanted to channel the new pool funds toward the voluntary hospitals because they feared the city would reduce its subsidy to HHC to offset pool fund gains. Accordingly, the distribution rules for the additional revenues from the bad debt and charity care pools provided relatively limited fiscal gains for the HHC.

In 1985, the state did not seek to continue its Medicare waiver, and in January of 1986 New York joined most other states in having its Medicare hospital payments made on the basis of diagnosis-related groups (DRGs). This was expected to benefit the state's hospitals, because DRG payments were estimated to be more generous than the allowable Medicare payments under NYPHRM. However, the state continued its restriction of per diem payments for other third parties and maintained the bad debt and charity care pool. The state regulatory system recently made a transition to per-case rather than per diem payments for third parties. As noted earlier, Governor Mario Cuomo proposed that the costs of graduate medical education and capital construction be shifted from a historical base to statewide discretionary pools.

The effect of the new, post-NYPHRM system on the municipal hospitals remains unclear. With respect to Medicare, which is only a small fraction of HHC revenues, short-run revenue losses are predicted because HHC costs are above the federal payment levels. Possible reductions in the indirect teaching cost allowance components of the DRG rates could lead to additional long-run revenue losses. Because the state's policies for transition to a per-case payment system for other third parties and possible changes in the distribution of bad debt and charity care pool funds have not yet been specified, the long-run outlook for HHC under the new state system is not clear.

*Regulating residencies.* The latest state regulatory initiative is to revise the scale and nature of graduate medical education in the state of New York. The health commissioner has declared, "I believe the time has come to regulate the quality, quantity and distribution of graduate medical education in New York State . . . I believe the State Health Department should have primary responsibility for this regulatory activity."[12] A special state advisory commission has recommended a 30 percent reduction in the number of residencies in the state, a greater proportion of primary care residencies, and sharp limits on the acceptance of foreign medical graduates in residency programs.[13] It is expected that the governor will seek authority to exercise some control over graduate medical education in the near future.

State regulation of residency positions could have significant implications for the HHC. Since the municipal facilities rely heavily on residents for services and in some instances rely primarily on foreign medical graduates to fill their residencies, regulations such as those proposed by the state advisory commission could force major changes in the way in which the HHC provides medical services. To date, the HHC has not devised any long-run plan to alter its medical staffing pattern.

**Overview of Policy Variables.** The foregoing history of the city of New York's policies for providing care to the poor and of the state of New York's regulatory policies can be summarized and related to the current situation by reviewing the principal policy decisions now shaping the municipal hospital system. The four policy variables identified in the preceding chapter — governance arrangements, financing, medical staffing patterns, and market strategy — provide the framework for this overview.

*Governance.* The board of the Health and Hospitals Corporation is able, in theory, to operate independently of municipal overhead agencies and regulations with respect to purchasing, staffing, and budgeting. In practice, however, its independence has varied over time. Currently, Mayor Edward I. Koch uses his appropriation and appointment powers to control HHC operations.

*Financing.* The HHC finances its operations with a combination of third-party collections and a local tax subsidy appropriated annually by the city. Third-party revenues consist principally of Medicaid collections, which as noted earlier have varied with state eligibility and reimbursement policies as well as the vigor of HHC collection efforts. In recent years, Medicaid collections have grown substantially and currently account for nearly one-half of all HHC revenues; the tax levy subsidy has averaged just below one-quarter of total HHC revenues (see Table 3.3). As discussed below, the HHC's relatively heavy reliance on tax levy funds has limited its ability to exercise political autonomy and has made the quality of its care and the efficiency with which that care is delivered largely dependent on the overall fiscal situation of the municipal government.

*Medical staffing.* The medical staff of HHC facilities is provided predominantly through affiliation contracts with teaching institutions. The affiliations are strong in the sense that affiliates control hiring for all medical staff positions, are responsible for all patient care, and play significant roles in determining the hospitals' service mix. As will be discussed below, these affiliation policies have improved quality of care at HHC hospitals by ensuring an abundant and well-trained physician staff; however, they also contribute to high costs and may limit the HHC's ability to carry out its basic mission of providing primary care to the city's poor.

*Market strategy.* The HHC has been and remains an institution strongly committed to serving the indigent. In times of fiscal stringency, when both Medicaid and tax levy funds have been in especially short supply, it has maintained access and not limited the volume of care provided to the poor, although quality of care has declined during those times because of lower spending and staffing levels. The HHC has made no major efforts to compete with private and voluntary hospitals for insured, middle-class constituencies. Rather, its policy is to endorse measures that promote access for the poor to voluntary as well as public facilities. Accordingly, HHC historically has reduced its scale of operations as overall utilization in the city has shifted toward the private sector.

## Trends in Performance

The performance of the HHC can be assessed in terms of its efficiency in providing services, the quality of its output, and the contribution its services make to providing access to care among the city's poor. The following sections assess these three categories—efficiency, quality, and access—in terms of both performance relative to other institutions and trends in performance over time.

## Efficiency

Efficiency is a relationship between input and output. Measuring the output of the HHC, as well as of other hospitals, is problematic because of variation in the types of service produced (inpatient versus outpatient), in the intensity of service within inpatient and outpatient categories, and in the quality of each type of service. Thus, analysis of efficiency must draw on a number of separate indicators.

One approach to assessing efficiency uses an output measure that standardizes for variation in product mix by combining inpatient admissions and outpatient services into a single unit of service, and calculates a cost per "adjusted admission" (see Table 3.6). In each year from 1979 to 1984 for which data are available, the HHC had a higher cost per adjusted admission than did hospitals in the rest of the state of New York and in the nation as a whole. During these years, the HHC's unit costs ranged between 33 and 51 percent higher than those of hospitals in the rest of the state and between 60 and 90 percent higher than those of hospitals nationwide.

The above measure of efficiency controls for variation in types (inpatient and outpatient) of service produced. However, it does not take into consideration other factors that affect the cost of services in an individual hospital, such as differences in wages, case mix, patient income and insurance, and physician practice patterns. A statistical model described in Chapter 7 takes these and other factors into account in explaining unit costs. This model permits a more refined assessment of efficiency by comparing actual HHC costs to those that would be predicted by the model after these other factors are taken into account.[14]

This analysis reveals that only two of the nine HHC hospitals for which data were available (Coney Island and Cumberland) had actual costs below their predicted costs, indicating relatively efficient performance for these two hospitals (see Table 3.7). Three other hospitals (Metropolitan, Kings County, and Bellevue) had actual costs up to 15 percent higher than their predicted costs. The remaining four HHC hospitals had actual costs more than 20 percent above predicted costs. Two of these four hospitals, Harlem and Bronx Municipal, had costs more than 40 percent higher than predicted in the model.

The relatively high unit costs at HHC facilities are related to apparently high staffing levels for nonphysician employees. The ratio of such workers to a standard work load measure (adjusted admissions)

## Table 3.6

## HHC Expenses per Adjusted Admission

|                        | *FY 1979* | *FY 1982* | *FY 1983* | *FY 1984* |
|------------------------|-----------|-----------|-----------|-----------|
| Bellevue               | $4,051    | $5,299    | $5,373    | $6,525    |
| Bronx Municipal        | 3,524     | 4,765     | 5,191     | 5,772     |
| City at Elmhurst       | 2,766     | 4,036     | 4,268     | 5,060     |
| Coney Island           | 2,470     | 3,225     | 3,648     | 4,000     |
| Harlem                 | 3,667     | 3,797     | 4,697     | 6,254     |
| Kings County           | 2,485     | 3,455     | 4,253     | 5,178     |
| Lincoln                | 3,287     | 3,336     | 3,491     | 3,696     |
| Metropolitan           | 2,668     | 4,188     | 4,683     | 5,599     |
| North Central Bronx    | 3,328     | 3,922     | 4,008     | 4,790     |
| Queens                 | 3,108     | 4,278     | 4,275     | NA        |
|                        |           |           |           |           |
| HHC average            | 3,103     | 4,080     | 4,423     | 5,247     |
| New York State average | 2,053     | 3,032     | 3,335     | 3,658     |
| United States average  | 1,631     | 2,493     | 2,776     | 2,934     |

Sources: Patient days and length of stay data from NYC Health and Hospitals Corporation, "Hospital Statistical Notes #1−1985, Hospital Care Facilities Data for the Fiscal Year 1984 in Comparison with the Fiscal Year 1983"; "Hospital Care Facilities Data for the Fiscal Year 1982 in Comparison with the Fiscal Year 1981"; "Hospital Statistical Notes #3−1981, Hospital Care Facilities Data for the Fiscal Year 1979." Expenditure data from Blue Cross and New York State, "Institutional Cost Report for Hospitals," FYs 1979, 1982, 1984, Worksheet C-3. Revenue data from Blue Cross and New York State, "Supplement to the Institutional Cost Report," FYs 1979, 1982, 1984, Exhibit I. Data for New York State and United States from American Hospital Association, *Hospital Statistics,* 1980, 1983, 1984, and 1985 editions, Tables 3 and 5c.

Note: Expenses per adjusted admission calculated as follows:

$$\left( \frac{\text{total expenses} \left( \frac{\text{inpatient revenue}}{\text{total patient revenue}} \right)}{\text{inpatient days}} \right) \text{average length of stay}$$

NA: Not available.

is significantly higher for HHC facilities than for most other community hospitals (see Table 3.8). In 1982, the HHC employed 10.2 full-time workers for every 100 adjusted admissions, well above the figures for other hospitals in the city (8.6) and all community hospitals in the 100 largest cities in the nation (8.4). Only two HHC hospitals had staff levels below those benchmarks−Greenpoint, which was in the process of closing in 1982, and Coney Island, which appears to be a relatively efficient hospital. The other HHC facilities had ratios ranging up to Bronx Municipal's high of 13.9.

Although HHC facilities are operated inefficiently in the sense that unit costs are higher than among comparable hospitals nationwide, the differences appear to have narrowed between 1979, when the HHC unit costs were 90 percent above the national average, and 1983,

## Table 3.7

## Operating Costs per Discharge
## for Municipal Hospitals, 1982

| Hospital | Predicted | Actual | Ratio | Variance in Standard Deviations |
|---|---|---|---|---|
| Coney Island | $4,915 | $4,130 | 0.84 | (0.80) |
| Cumberland | 3,103 | 2,768 | 0.89 | (0.52) |
| Kings County | 3,856 | 4,320 | 1.12 | 0.53 |
| Greenpoint | 2,821 | 3,612 | 1.28 | 1.14 |
| Metropolitan | 3,718 | 4,265 | 1.15 | 0.64 |
| Bellevue | 4,192 | 4,670 | 1.11 | 0.50 |
| Elmhurst | 3,858 | 4,784 | 1.24 | 1.00 |
| Harlem | 4,015 | 5,620 | 1.40 | 1.57 |
| Bronx Municipal | 3,855 | 5,547 | 1.44 | 1.70 |

Source: Calculations by authors based on regression equation presented in Chapter 7.

## Table 3.8

## Staff-to-Work-Load Measures for HHC
## Facilities and Other Groups of Hospitals, 1982

| Hospital | Full-Time Nonphysician Employees per 100 Adjusted Admissions* |
|---|---|
| North Central Bronx | 11.7 |
| Coney Island | 7.4 |
| Greenpoint | 6.6 |
| Kings County | 9.1 |
| Queens | 8.9 |
| Bellevue | 13.6 |
| Bronx Municipal | 13.9 |
| Harlem | 9.3 |
| Lincoln | 8.9 |
| Metropolitan | 12.0 |
| Elmhurst | 10.0 |
| HHC average | 10.2 |
| All other New York City community hospitals | 8.6 |
| All community hospitals in 100 largest cities | 8.4 |

Source: Data from 1982 joint AHA–Urban Institute survey.

*Adjusted admissions are as defined in Table 3.6.

when the gap had dropped to 59 percent (see Table 3.6). This trend probably began in the mid-1970s when inflation-adjusted HHC expenditures stopped growing, in contrast to the experience nationally. However, the trend toward greater efficiency at HHC was reversed in 1984, when the gap between HHC costs and those elsewhere widened. Until more recent data are available and analyzed, this should be interpreted as a cautionary sign rather than as a turning point in HHC's record of improved relative efficiency in the early 1980s.

## Quality of Care

Assessing the quality of health care is also a difficult task. There are few widely agreed-upon standards of quality, and data relating to many suggested criteria often are unavailable. Nonetheless, available evidence points to three conclusions about the quality of care in HHC facilities.

First, HHC facilities generally provide services that meet standards of minimum adequacy. This, at least, is suggested by the fact that all HHC facilities are accredited by the Joint Commission, in each case for the maximum three years.

Moreover, it appears that the quality of HHC services is, on average, more than minimally adequate. The Joint Commission review process involves reporting on 24 functional subject areas (most broadly divided into safety, support, and medical services), each of which is divided into component parts or standards. Deviations from these standards are reported in the Joint Commission findings as recommendations to hospitals, calling for correction. A study of these reports from 1980 to 1982 compared public and voluntary hospitals in New York City in 11 functional areas deemed representative of the 24 areas for all HHC hospitals and for two categories of nonprofit institution: hospitals with fewer than 400 beds and those with more than 400 beds.[15] Overall, the HHC had a mean of 37.8 recommendations per hospital, compared to 42.7 for nonprofit hospitals with fewer than 400 beds and 46.9 for those voluntary institutions with more than 400 beds. For 9 of the 11 functions HHC hospitals had fewer recommendations than did each of the two groups of nonprofit institutions. Based on these results it appears that the HHC hospitals offer comparable, if not better, services than typical voluntary facilities.

Additional evidence of more than minimally adequate care is the relatively abundant supply of physicians available for patient care at HHC facilities. A study using 1983 data assessed the supply of physicians at HHC hospitals by comparing the volume of services provided to the number of full-time-equivalent physicians.[16] For HHC hospitals as a group, each physician performed work equivalent to 3,484 outpatient visits per year. This is well below a federally established standard of 4,200. This is accounted for primarily by the large amount of physician time spent supervising resident care, widely viewed as a sign of high quality medical care.

Although HHC facilities meet minimal standards for JCAH accreditation and have more than adequate physician staff, there are widely acknowledged qualitative deficiencies. Most frequently cited is a shortage of skilled nursing personnel. A study of HHC nurse staffing levels compared available nursing hours with the hours required by industry standards and revealed serious shortcomings.[17] In fiscal year 1982, available nursing hours equaled only 79 percent of the recommended total; in fiscal year 1984 the percentage was somewhat higher but still only 82 percent. Although aspects of hospital care other than physician and nurse staffing have not been systematically studied, there is a widely held perception that at HHC hospitals some support services, such as housekeeping and food services, fall below standards prevailing in the local voluntary sector.

A second important point is that quality of care varies widely among the individual hospitals within the HHC system. On most dimensions of quality, some facilities perform quite well while others evidence serious deficiencies.

The variation in quality was evident in the study of nurse staffing cited above. For example, in fiscal year 1984, when the average number of nursing hours available was 82 percent of the industry standard, 2 facilities actually exceeded the standard (Elmhurst and the newly opened Woodhull); 3 (Harlem, Kings, and Queens) met at least 90 percent of the standard; the remaining 10 facilities were below 90 percent of the standard, including 3 hospitals (Gouverneur, Goldwater, and Lincoln) that were below two-thirds of the standard.

Variation in quality also was evident in an analysis of the frequency of "sentinel events" at HHC facilities.[18] As applied to inpatient hospital care, the sentinel event approach identifies unnecessary deaths occurring during hospitalizations. Such deaths were found to occur in 17 of every 1,000 cases in the study group within HHC facilities in 1982. However, the rate per 1,000 cases varied from 6 at North Central Bronx to 25 at Harlem Hospital.

Finally, the variation in quality of care is reflected in another frequently used indicator — foreign medical graduates filling residency positions (see Table 3.9). For all HHC facilities combined, graduates of U.S. medical schools filled about 65 percent of the 846 first-year openings in 1985. However, the proportion varied widely among HHC institutions and their affiliates. At Bronx Municipal, North Central

Bronx, Queens General, and Bellevue, over 90 percent of the openings were filled by U.S. medical school graduates. In contrast, at Woodhull only 1 of the 29 openings was filled by a U.S. medical school graduate. The shares at Lincoln and Coney Island were only slightly better than one-third; the share was less than one-half at Kings County and Elmhurst; and Metropolitan and Harlem filled only 52 percent and 57 percent, respectively, of their residency openings with U.S. medical graduates.

A third general point about quality is that it appears to have deteriorated during the post-fiscal crisis period but improved some-what since 1980. The basis for this conclusion is limited to indirect inferences from aggregate data. In the 1975–80 period, the HHC suf-fered significant reductions in available resources. Its revenues were constrained by state Medicaid policies and limited tax levy appropria-tions. As a result, sizable staff reductions were required. The number of corporate staff, including affiliate employees, fell from a 1975 high of 49,080 to a 1980 low of 40,431 (see Table 3.4). While some gains in efficiency were achieved during this period, the loss of nearly one of every five employees—at a time when the volume of admissions was sustained—also adversely affected quality. Since the losses were pre-dominantly among nonphysician staff, the types of quality reduction were related to standards of nursing care and support services rather than to direct medical care.

The more than 52 percent increase in budget and roughly 10 percent increase in staff since 1980—with little change in service volume—have probably permitted quality improvements. These gains are reflected in the expansion of nursing staff, the medical records initiative, the ambulatory care initiative, and other programmatic improvements described earlier. In this sense, quality of care improved at HHC since 1980.

### Access

New York City offers relatively good access to necessary medical care for the indigent population. Comparative data for the nation's 100 largest cities (presented more fully in Chapter 7) reveal that the num-ber of adjusted admissions per 100 poor residents in New York City (30 per 100) is somewhat higher than would be predicted based on its market characteristics (28 per 100).

Within New York City there is generally equal access to some form of care for both poor and nonpoor residents. Survey data suggest that approximately equal shares of poor and nonpoor adults see a physician at least once during the year (78 percent versus 79 percent).[19]

## Table 3.9

## Medical Graduates Filling First-Year Residency Positions at HHC Facilities, July 1985

| Affiliate/Hospital | U.S. Graduates | | U.S. Foreign Graduates | | Alien Foreign Graduates | | Total | |
|---|---|---|---|---|---|---|---|---|
| | No. | % | No. | % | No. | % | No. | % |
| Columbia/Harlem | 37 | 56.9 | 4 | 6.2 | 24 | 36.9 | 65 | 100.0 |
| CIPC/Coney Island | 19 | 38.8 | 9 | 18.4 | 21 | 42.9 | 49 | 100.0 |
| Downstate/Kings County | 55 | 45.8 | 28 | 23.3 | 37 | 30.8 | 120 | 100.0 |
| Einstein/Bronx Municipal | 89 | 94.7 | 1 | 1.1 | 4 | 4.3 | 94 | 100.0 |
| Montefiore/North Central Bronx | 88 | 94.6 | 2 | 2.2 | 3 | 3.2 | 93 | 100.0 |
| LIJ/Queens General | 78 | 90.7 | 7 | 8.1 | 1 | 1.2 | 86 | 100.0 |
| Mt. Sinai/Elmhurst | 41 | 48.2 | 27 | 31.8 | 17 | 20.0 | 85 | 100.0 |
| NYMC/Lincoln | 22 | 33.8 | 20 | 30.8 | 23 | 35.4 | 65 | 100.0 |
| NYMC/Metropolitan | 34 | 52.3 | 8 | 12.3 | 23 | 35.4 | 65 | 100.0 |
| NYU/Bellevue | 89 | 93.7 | 3 | 3.2 | 3 | 3.2 | 95 | 100.0 |
| MAWPC/Woodhull | 1 | 3.4 | 6 | 20.7 | 22 | 75.9 | 29 | 100.0 |
| Total | 553 | 65.4 | 115 | 13.6 | 178 | 21.0 | 846 | 100.0 |

Source: Unpublished data from Vice-President for Medical Affairs, New York City Health and Hospitals Corporation.

Some 13 percent of poor adults and 6 percent of poor children are hospitalized, compared to only 9 percent of nonpoor adults and 4 percent of nonpoor children. This differential in hospitalization rates does not take into account differences in health status, but it suggests relatively good access for the poor. Troubling, however, is the fact that substantially fewer poor children than nonpoor children see a doctor each year (81 percent versus 91 percent); but in both cases the proportion is relatively high.

The HHC plays a major role in ensuring a high degree of access to medical care for poor residents of New York City, as evidenced by recent estimates of the volume and cost of uncompensated care by all hospitals in New York City. Between 1981 and 1983, all hospitals in the city, combined, provided between $450 million and $516 million in uncompensated care. The HHC hospitals accounted for over one-half of those annual totals, and as much as 58 percent in 1982.[20] The HHC hospitals are also particularly important to Medicaid recipients in the city. With only 18 percent of the general care beds, HHC hospitals account for about 39 percent of all Medicaid discharges in the city.[21]

Although the mission of the HHC is to provide access to necessary medical care for all New Yorkers regardless of income, it devotes the overwhelming share of its resources to those with Medicaid coverage and those medically indigent with no insurance coverage (frequently dubbed "self-pay" or, more accurately, "no pay" patients). These patients account for almost 66 percent of all HHC inpatient days, 71 percent of the corporation's outpatient department visits, and 79 percent of its emergency room visits (see Table 3.10).

Precise data on the volume of care provided to the poor by HHC in recent years are not available, but nothing suggests there was any change in the corporation's basic commitment to the poor even during the 1975–80 period when some inpatient facilities were closed. These changes led to higher occupancy rates rather than to reduced inpatient admissions (see Table 3.11). During the 1980s, the state's support to voluntary hospitals for uncompensated care, through NYPHRM, may have facilitated a shift of utilization among the indigent from municipal to voluntary hospitals. Whether or not this has occurred, the basic fact that the HHC's primary mission is to serve the city's poor remains unaltered.

## Table 3.10

## Expected Source of Payment for
## Inpatient and Ambulatory Care Services at HHC Facilities
## (percentage distribution)

| | |
|---|---:|
| Inpatient days | |
| Medicaid | 45.4% |
| Medicare | 22.7 |
| Blue Cross | 8.9 |
| Commercial insurance | 2.7 |
| Other[a] | 20.3 |
| Total | 100.0% |
| Outpatient department visits | |
| Medicaid | 36.0% |
| Medicare | 18.2 |
| Blue Cross | 0.7 |
| Other insurance | 0.6 |
| Self-pay | 35.1 |
| Other[b] | 9.4 |
| Total | 100.0% |
| Emergency room visits | |
| Medicaid | 24.0% |
| Medicare | 5.5 |
| Blue Cross | 9.9 |
| Other insurance | 2.6 |
| Self-pay | 54.6 |
| Other[b] | 3.0 |
| Total | 100.0% |

Sources: Inpatient data for 1982 from annual report of the New York State Department of Health, Statewide and Research Corporation Systems; outpatient and emergency room data for third quarter of 1983 from United Hospital Fund, Patient Origin Information System.

[a]Includes workers' compensation, self-pay, and uncompensated care.

[b]Free care.

## Governance

### Current Arrangements

As described earlier, operation of the municipal hospitals has been the responsibility of the HHC since 1970. Five members of its 16-member board are municipal officials who serve at the discretion of the mayor as ex officio members: the health services administrator, the health commissioner, the commissioner of mental health and mental retardation, the human resources administrator, and a deputy mayor. The health services administrator also is designated by statute as the

## Table 3.11

## Occupancy Rates in HHC Facilities

| Hospital | Overall Occupancy Rate, % | | | General Care Occupancy Rate, % | | |
|---|---|---|---|---|---|---|
| | *1975* | *1980* | *1984* | *1975* | *1980* | *1984* |
| Bellevue | 76 | 85 | 87 | 75 | 85 | 87 |
| Bronx Municipal | 75 | 80 | 77 | 78 | 79 | 77 |
| Coler | 89 | 88 | 93 | NA | NA | NA |
| Coney Island | 71 | 92 | 92 | 82 | 93 | 92 |
| Cumberland | 81 | 71 | C | 81 | 70 | C |
| Elmhurst | 77 | 79 | 86 | 71 | 72 | 85 |
| Fordham | 81 | C | C | 81 | C | C |
| Francis Delafield | 61 | C | C | 61 | C | C |
| Goldwater | 82 | 95 | 96 | 71 | NA | NA |
| Gouverneur | 61 | 96 | 99 | 64 | NA | NA |
| Greenpoint | 85 | 74 | C | 85 | 74 | C |
| Harlem | 81 | 76 | 83 | 78 | 78 | 83 |
| Kings County | 77 | 76 | 82 | 76 | 76 | 82 |
| Lincoln | 81 | 86 | 94 | 81 | 86 | 94 |
| Metropolitan | 76 | 79 | 84 | 76 | 75 | 84 |
| Morrisania | 76 | C | C | 76 | C | C |
| North Central Bronx | NO | 87 | 84 | NO | 87 | 84 |
| Queens | 74 | 67 | 79 | 73 | 69 | 79 |
| Sea View | 94 | 98 | 100 | 96 | NA | 100 |
| Sydenham | 67 | 81 | C | 68 | 83 | C |
| Woodhull | NO | NO | 89 | NO | NO | 89 |
| Total | 79 | 82 | 87 | 73 | 82 | 87 |

Sources: NYC Health and Hospitals Corporation, "Hospital Statistical Notes #3 — 1981"; "Hospital Statistical Notes #4 — 1978, Profile Statistical Data, Corporate Hospitals, 1973-1977"; "Hospital Statistical Notes #1 — 1985."

NA: Not applicable (institution does not have general care beds).

C: Closed.

NO: Institution had not yet opened at that date.

chairman of the board. Ten additional members are appointed by the mayor for five-year terms, but five of these mayoral appointees are designated by the city council. The sixteenth member of the board is its president, who serves as chief operating officer and is selected by the other 15 members. The president does not have a stationary term of office and may be hired and fired at the discretion of the board.

Although the board was intended to be semiautonomous, it has come under close mayoral control in recent years. Mayor Koch, first elected in 1977, campaigned with the position that the municipal hospitals should be a mayoral department. Although he has not proposed legislation to change the formal status of the HHC board, he has used his appointment and budget powers to achieve the same result. Since being elected, Mayor Koch has had the opportunity to appoint new members to all 10 appointive positions. These members were chosen, in part, because they are sensitive to the mayor's desire to control HHC activities closely.

All major HHC decisions are reviewed by the mayor or his staff, including senior appointments, budget modifications, and contracts. Since the first deputy mayor, Stanley Brezenoff, is a former HHC president, there is a strong working knowledge of HHC operations within the mayor's office and close coordination between the board and city hall.

Internally, HHC programs are operated through 11 acute care hospitals, four separate long-term care facilities, and two independently managed neighborhood family care centers. In addition, HHC hospitals manage three other NFCCs and numerous satellite programs. The executive directors of the hospitals and the administrators of the NFCCs are selected formally by the president, but these appointments are reviewed informally by the mayor, as implied by the discussion above. Each of the hospitals is affiliated with a private facility for the provision of medical staff, and the management of the institution is conducted in cooperation with a medical board and an advisory community board.

In general, there is strong central control over the management of individual institutions. There are corporate vice-presidents or units for finance, management information systems, medical affairs, nursing, planning, legal affairs, public relations, and other major functions. Executive directors submit frequent periodic reports to the central office on their activities. In addition, the central office oversees the affiliated private institutions' performance in providing medical staff.

## Implications of Governance Arrangements

The 1970 shift in governance arrangements from a mayoral agency to a semiautonomous public benefit corporation presumed three beneficial results. First, improvements were anticipated in quality of care because HHC would have increased incentives to collect third-party revenues and, thus, more money to spend for services. Second, greater efficiency would result from managerial freedom from centralized personnel, purchasing, and budget control imposed by city-wide agencies. Third, decentralization, achieved through subsidiary corporations that would manage individual facilities, was expected to create greater consumer responsiveness.

The creation of the HHC was followed by a five-year period

during which the board operated with some autonomy and realized certain of its expectations. The initial arrangements provided strong incentives for the HHC to increase third-party collections. In addition, greater flexibility in salary and other personnel rules facilitated recruitment of higher quality, upper-level managers than would have been possible under civil service arrangements.

However, this period also was characterized by fiscal instability resulting from weak links to the municipal budgetary process. Because the HHC board was seeking to maximize revenues, it fought with the city's OMB over estimates of likely third-party revenues and the corollary, the size of the needed subsidy. This often left the agency in an uncertain fiscal position with respect to its subsidy, which, in turn, hampered improvements in service delivery and planning.

The state emergency financial control board, created in 1975, required better financial planning between the board and city, thereby limiting HHC's autonomy. The political preferences and policies of Mayor Koch reinforced the fiscally induced overhead controls and made mayoral domination easier when the fiscal crisis ended.

One consequence, implemented without change in the legal governance structure, has been to make HHC's finances less contentious and more stable. Moreover, the loss in political autonomy does not appear to have weakened HHC's incentives to strengthen third-party collections, since such revenues have increased with mayoral control without being offset by reduced subsidies. Thus, reversion to mayoral control has not hurt HHC finances — quite the contrary.

If HHC's governance has not attained the independence from city hall envisaged by its creators, neither has its management evolved in the decentralized way that was envisaged. The HHC remains an organization with fairly tight central control over individual facilities. Labor negotiations are conducted along with those for other city agencies; affiliation contracts are negotiated by the HHC central office rather than by individual hospitals; hospital budgets and their administration are subject to central HHC review and, to some extent, to review by the city's OMB. Some hospital directors have political bases that permit them to bypass HHC controls occasionally, but in general the routine operations of hospital management are no more free of overhead control than are operations in mayoral agencies.

In summary, the formal change in the legal governance structure that was fashioned in 1970 has not had a strong, direct impact on efficiency, quality, or access. The relative autonomy of the initial five-year period was set aside for financial and political reasons after 1975. Whatever changes have occurred in performance reflect other policies, not the structure of the HHC's governance.

## Financing

The financing of the HHC can be described in terms of the process used to determine and administer its budget and its outcomes in the form of actual revenues and expenditures. These topics are considered below.

### Current Arrangements

The HHC's budget process is aligned closely with New York City's. The HHC budget cycle begins in the summer preceding the start of the fiscal year. At that time, central office officials send guidelines to the directors of each facility for preparation of their budget requests. The guidelines provide common assumptions for inflationary increases in expenditure requirements and indicate programmatic areas that have priority for new resources. Executive directors are expected to justify budget requests in terms of projected changes in work load and of any new initiatives that would be undertaken in the priority areas.

In the fall, negotiations take place between the executive directors and central office personnel in order to arrive at a corporate budget to be submitted to the OMB in November. The HHC budget submission justifies increases from the previous year for inflation, changes in projected work load, and new initiatives. The budget submission also presents estimates of revenue sources, including, in particular, the subsidy requested of the city.

In December, HHC and OMB officials negotiate a budget to be included in the financial plan that the mayor is required to submit to the Financial Control Board (FCB) in January. Negotiations tend to focus on the appropriate third-party revenue targets for HHC and the size of the city's subsidy. The OMB generally follows mayoral directions in targeting any new HHC resources to priority programs.

Between January and March, the mayor's proposals (for all city agencies as well as the HHC) are reviewed by the state fiscal monitors and by the local legislative bodies, the city council and the board of estimate. The fiscal monitors are concerned only with the reasonableness of the revenue and expenditure estimates; they search for significant unidentified risks in the form of expenditure increases that may not be provided for or revenues that may be overestimated.

In late April the mayor is required to submit an executive budget that provides detailed appropriations for all agencies, including the HHC, for the coming fiscal year. At the same time the mayor generally submits to the FCB a revised financial plan, which also includes a budget for the HHC. These budgets again are reviewed by the fiscal monitors, and the budget for the city must be approved by the board of estimate and the city council. Reviews by the board of estimate and city council are less technical and focus more on the priorities in the mayor's budget. In general, the city council has been less sympathetic to requests for additional funds for the HHC than for police and education. Thus, in the joint legislative hearings the HHC must typically defend the budget increases previously approved by the OMB and the mayor. Final negotiations between the mayor and the legislative bodies typically take place late in June, when both a budget and a revised financial plan must be approved before the start of the new fiscal year on July 1.

The HHC administers its own budget but does so under close scrutiny by the OMB. The HHC is responsible for collections from patients and third parties and has its own payment systems for payroll and purchases. These collection and payment systems are either directly administered or closely supervised by the HHC central office, which reports periodically to the OMB on collections and expenditures. Based on these reports, the OMB allocates cash transfers to the HHC in accord with the approved sum for the annual city subsidy. The HHC finance unit, in cooperation with the OMB, also submits quarterly reports to the FCB to indicate compliance with the approved financial plan. Modifications to the plan must be approved by the FCB; if modifications require increases in the subsidy, they must be approved by the city council.

The foregoing procedures resulted in total HHC operating expenditures of nearly $2 billion in fiscal year 1985 (see Table 3.3). Of the total, 14 percent was devoted to affiliation contracts and 68 percent was for compensation of the HHC's nearly 44,000 employees.

Revenues of the HHC are broadly divided between collections from third parties, which accounted for about 70 percent of the total in 1985, and the subsidy from the city. The largest source of third-party revenues is Medicaid, which accounts for about 46 percent of all revenues. Smaller sums are received from Medicare (14 percent), Blue Cross (5 percent), and other sources (5 percent).

The third-party payer mix varies between inpatient and outpatient services (see Table 3.10). Medicaid is the expected source of payment for over 45 percent of all inpatient days but for only about 36 percent of outpatient department (OPD) visits and 24 percent of emergency room (ER) visits. Medicare accounts for about one-fifth of the inpatient days and OPD visits, but for only about 6 percent of ER visits. Blue Cross payments cover slightly less than 10 percent of inpatient days and ER visits, but virtually no OPD services. Self-pay patients, who account for most of the HHC's bad debts, represent about 20 percent of inpatient days, more than 35 percent of OPD visits, and nearly 55 percent of ER visits.

The city's subsidy to the HHC consists of both cash payments and in-kind services provided by the city. The in-kind contributions include utilities provided by the city's general services administration to HHC buildings, sanitation services for the hospitals, and rental of certain equipment. In addition, the city makes payments to employee pension funds and pays workers' compensation fund contributions on behalf of the HHC. These in-kind services and payments account for about one-half of the city's subsidy. The remainder, cash transfers, includes a larger direct cash subsidy and payments under contracts with the city's Department of Mental Health for psychiatric services provided at corporate facilities.

The trend in recent years has been toward reduced tax levy support and greater third-party, notably Medicaid, revenues (see Table 3.3). Between fiscal years 1980 and 1984, the city subsidy fell from 37 to 24 percent of total revenues, while Medicaid revenues increased from 34 to 48 percent.

## Implications of Financing Arrangements

The dominant fact of current HHC finances is strong reliance on local tax subsidies and a consequent strong role for local public officials in the budgetary and programmatic decisions of the HHC. Three important consequences flow from this combination of fiscal and political links.

First, the financing arrangements tie the programmatic changes in HHC's operations to the overall fiscal condition of the city. Despite its access to substantial third-party revenues that it collects independently, the HHC's total expenditures are set through a budgetary process that strongly reflects the overall resources available to the city as a whole. City funds are a "last dollar" appropriation that is adjusted to reflect total revenues expected from other sources; therefore, the HHC budget is, in the end, determined by the size of the city subsidy.

The dependence on local subsidies also influences the potential trade-off between access and quality of care. Staff reductions during the 1975–80 period reduced the quality of care but maintained access; when resources grew during the 1980s, they were allocated primarily to quality improvements rather than expanded access. In other words, under the current financing and governance arrangements, policy adjustments to variations in available resources resulting from changing municipal financial conditions primarily affect the quality of care rather than access to care.

Finally, the HHC's dependence on local subsidies has not been a disincentive for efficiency improvements. The HHC was able to narrow the "efficiency gap" between itself and other hospitals both during retrenchment in the second half of the 1970s and during growth in the 1980s, at least through 1983. These gains were made possible by the pressures exerted by municipal oversight agencies and by the demands of elected leaders to improve performance, rather than from any "businesslike" practices that allegedly flow from more political autonomy. The strong political and fiscal dependence of HHC on politicians experiencing constrained resources appears to have contributed to relative efficiency gains — again, a relationship that would not have been expected by many theorists or, for that matter, by the proponents of HHC's creation nearly two decades ago.

## Medical Staffing

The dominant HHC medical staffing pattern is affiliation with teaching institutions. However, the nature of the affiliations differs, depending largely on the extent to which the affiliate integrates resident teaching at its home facility and its municipal facility.

### Current Arrangements

The closest affiliations normally prevail at geographically adjacent (and in some cases physically attached) facilities: Montefiore Hospital and North Bronx General; Einstein College and Bronx Municipal; Downstate Medical College and Kings County; and New York University (NYU) and Bellevue. In addition, NYU provides staff to nearby Goldwater and Gouverneur Hospitals.

New York Medical College is the affiliate of three municipal institutions — Lincoln Hospital in the Bronx, Metropolitan Hospital in Manhattan, and Coler Hospital, a long-term care facility on Roosevelt Island. Although New York Medical College recently moved its home facilities to Westchester County, it retains close ties to Lincoln in particular. The controversy surrounding proposals (now withdrawn) to close Metropolitan Hospital has made it difficult to attract residents to that municipal hospital in recent years. The college does not maintain residencies at Coler and uses attending staff to provide medical care.

Long Island Jewish Hospital is the affiliate for Queens General. It is located a few miles away but maintains closely integrated residency programs at both institutions. Harlem Hospital and its affiliate, Columbia University's College of Physicians and Surgeons, are close geographically but do not have well-integrated residency training for most specialties. Mt. Sinai Hospital in Manhattan is the affiliate for Elmhurst Hospital in Queens, but there is limited integration of residency training in this instance too.

The two remaining general care hospitals, Coney Island and Woodhull in Brooklyn, are affiliated with independent nonprofit physician groups that provide attending staff and supervise the relatively small number of residents at each municipal facility. In addition, there are academic affiliations involving no financial payments between Maimonidies Hospital and Coney Island and between Downstate Medical College and Woodhull.

While the closeness of relationships between voluntary hospitals and their municipal affiliates varies, the voluntaries all play a major role in the operation of the public hospitals. Under the affiliation contracts, the voluntaries are responsible for selecting all medical staff. (Physicians hired by HHC must be approved by the teaching institution.) In addition, the medical staff play a strong role in institutional decisions regarding service mix and the allocation of beds to competing services.

## Implications of Staffing Arrangements

The general policy of securing medical staff through contracts with affiliated teaching institutions has important implications for the quality and cost of care at HHC facilities. The teaching programs add to HHC costs, both through direct supervision changes and through indirect costs resulting from additional tests, more extensive diagnostic procedures, and more intensive treatment for the sickest patients. Coney Island Hospital, the major exception to HHC's policy of affiliating with a teaching hospital, has relatively low unit costs.

Another important financial implication of HHC's reliance on affiliates for medical staff is the consequent exclusion of privately insured patients from HHC facilities. Again with the exception of Coney Island Hospital, HHC does not permit its medical staff to bill separately for medical services but rather obtains payment for medical services through an "all-inclusive" per diem rate.[22] This provides little incentive for physicians to admit their privately insured patients to HHC facilities. Accordingly, affiliate staff members generally limit municipal admissions to indigent patients served in the outpatient departments of the municipal and voluntary institutions. Thus, HHC's policy limits its access to privately insured patients, which significantly affects its payer mix.

While expensive, the affiliation arrangements are generally recognized as having contributed significantly to improved quality of care at municipal facilities. At the time the affiliation contracts were initiated, physicians were in short supply; the contracts have helped ensure adequate physician supply at municipal facilities, as the figures on physician staff levels cited earlier indicate.

However, the contribution of the affiliation arrangements to quality of care varies widely among municipal facilities. Not all affiliates are attractive to physicians, particularly to graduates of U.S. medical schools. The variation in quality, inferred from the share of U.S. medical graduates described earlier (see Table 3.9), is related to the performance of the voluntary affiliate. Most of the institutions with close affiliation relationships are relatively successful in attracting U.S. medical graduates to their municipal affiliates: NYU, Montefiore, and Einstein are examples. In contrast, those institutions with weaker ties to their municipal affiliates are less able to secure U.S. medical graduates for their municipal facilities: Columbia and Mt. Sinai are illustrative. There are exceptions to this (notably Downstate and Kings County), but in general, the affiliation relationships that produce the best quality of care for the municipal facilities are those in which the two institutions are well integrated.

Although affiliation contracts benefit medical care in the municipal hospitals, there is general agreement that they divide operational authority within the municipal system and thus weaken hospital management. Since affiliation contracts are negotiated and monitored by HHC's central office rather than by hospital directors, the affiliates are not accountable to the institutions they are intended to serve. A further complication is that some affiliation contracts cover nonphysicians, who are represented by a different union than the one representing municipal hospital employees. Thus, voluntary hospital employees may work in municipal facilities for supervisors located elsewhere, and side by side with municipal hospital employees represented by a different union and working under different collective bargaining contracts. This situation limits the authority of municipal hospital managers and complicates labor-management relations.

Another set of problems with the affiliation relationships involves the fit between the programmatic needs of the teaching institutions and those of the municipal hospitals. The principal mission of the municipal hospitals is to provide services to the city's indigent population, which needs primary medical care (often best provided on an outpatient basis) and relatively routine inpatient procedures. The research and teaching mission of the affiliates, however, causes them to place high priority on specialized care that utilizes complex procedures. The adverse consequences include use of scarce resources for expensive specialized equipment, maintenance of a relatively large number of residencies at municipal hospitals in medical specialties rather than primary care, and organization of outpatient services into highly specialized clinics rather than more comprehensive arrangements that would simplify care of patients with multiple illnesses. Teaching and research concerns dominate because HHC has no alternative source of physician supply and has, therefore, limited bargaining power over the affiliates.

## Market Strategy

Throughout HHC's history the primary mission of the municipal hospitals has remained constant—to serve the indigent who lack access to other providers. The HHC has sought to execute this mission by providing care of comparable quality to that in the private sector; but the HHC has sought neither to displace the private sector as a source of care nor to compete for privately insured patients.

### Current Policy

The role of the HHC in providing care to the poor is evident in its market share for various types of services and patients. As noted earlier, the HHC accounts for about one-fifth of all general care beds in New York City. Using this benchmark, HHC accounts for disproportionately large shares of inpatient care to Medicaid patients and to so-called self-pay patients (39 percent each). Indigent patients account for about two-thirds of all HHC inpatient days. In contrast, the HHC cares for about 10 percent of all Blue Cross patients in the city, and this group represents less than 9 percent of HHC's total inpatient days. The HHC also provides a disproportionately large share of citywide OPD visits (46 percent) and ER visits (40 percent).

### Implications of Current Policy

The HHC's basic mission, serving the indigent, has a strong influence on its performance. As noted earlier, the HHC was obliged to trade quality for access when its budget was constrained, and more recently, with growing resources, funds were used to upgrade primary care rather than to expand the scope of services or compete for privately insured patients.

The implications of the HHC's market strategy for efficiency are more difficult to isolate. Resources available to the HHC depend on fiscal conditions more than on the size or needs of the patient population. When budgets are tight and demand increases, unit costs fall, although whether this reflects greater efficiency or lower quality is difficult to determine. During recent years, quality has improved and unit costs have increased more slowly than the national average.

## Summary and Future Outlook

The HHC's performance in the early 1980s suggests that the governance, staffing, and financing policies that have evolved since its creation in 1970 have served it reasonably well. In a period when social welfare programs were under close scrutiny, the HHC secured new resources, narrowed the efficiency gap between its operations and those of other hospitals, upgraded aspects of the quality of its care, and maintained access for the city's poor. Suggestions for altering HHC policies should rest on an understanding of these accomplishments and the institutional arrangements that support them.

The accomplishments of HHC derive from an effective fit between its basic mission of serving the poor and its governance and finance arrangements. This mission has strong political support in New York City, at least relative to the national mood and to such commitments in other major cities. Consequently, there are few tensions between the HHC board and the city's elected leaders; the latter provide political and financial support for the former. State policies too have contributed to HHC's accomplishments, particularly increased Medicaid funding and the additional support provided for indigent care through the bad debt and charity care fund.

These complementary relationships in mission, governance, and financing arrangements seem likely to continue in the future. Given its history, New York is likely to remain a city where residents and voters maintain political support for ensuring access to adequate medical care for the poor. The historical argument — improved efficiency — for seeking greater autonomy from political control does not seem relevant in the New York City case. The relative efficiency of HHC operations realized in recent years occurred because of reduced political autonomy; independence from municipal civil service and purchasing regulations is available without political autonomy.

The major obstacle to greater efficiency is related to medical staffing policies rather than to arrangements for governance and financing. Affiliation with teaching institutions contributes to added costs, but this policy can be changed without altering governance or financing arrangements.

The combination of strong political ties between municipal officials and the HHC board and a financing system that permits municipal officials to determine the overall size of the HHC budget means that HHC's fate is closely tied to the city's fiscal condition. The city of New York appears to be in reasonably good financial condition, and the state also seems able and willing to maintain and even enhance its Medicaid program and the bad debt and charity care pools. Despite the recent growth in hospital occupancy rates traced largely to AIDS patients and psychiatric patients, the fiscal outlook is further improved by widely recognized longer-term trends toward reduced demand for inpatient hospital care, which will lower total medical care expenditures. Both lengths of stay and admission rates are expected to continue to fall with the state's shift to a per-case payment system, as utilization review procedures are strengthened, as HMOs obtain a larger enrollment, and as state regulatory authority is used to reduce the overall bed capacity and the level of graduate medical education. Thus, relative to demand, resources for medical care to the poor are likely to be increasing.

As demand for care declines over the longer term, it is likely that the voluntary sector will increase its market share among the indigent population. In order to maintain current physical plant and capital equipment and retain specialized programs, voluntary institutions will seek a larger share of the declining total market. This includes greater numbers and proportions of Medicaid patients and the uninsured. Given a continued state commitment to reasonable Medicaid rates and a pool of funds for uncompensated care, the voluntary sector should be able to increase its market share among the indigent without substantial adverse fiscal consequences. The implication of these expected trends for the HHC is that the corporation will be able to shrink its bed capacity and its operating expenditures without sacrificing its mission as a last-resort provider.

The major potential misfit between current policies and future conditions is in the area of medical staffing. A number of developments suggest that alternatives to the affiliation arrangements may be both feasible and desirable. First, the growing number of physicians nationally and locally has made it easier for all types of institutions to recruit medical staff. In most specialities it is no longer difficult to recruit well-qualified younger physicians at reasonable levels of compensation. Second, state regulation of graduate medical education, which is likely, will mean reduced numbers of residencies and greater proportions of residencies in primary care specialties. The reduced number of residencies and the accompanying restrictions on recruitment of foreign medical graduates may make some residency programs in some of the municipal hospitals no longer viable. This could effectively eliminate the possibility of teaching affiliations for those hospitals that do not currently have high quality residency programs. On the other hand, the greater emphasis on primary care specialties within the network of graduate medical education programs will make the municipal hospitals desirable sites for such residencies. Because the HHC's service mission is strongly weighted toward provision of primary care to the indigent, municipal facilities have a large patient population suited to primary care residencies. Thus, the proposed types of regulation may make at least some parts of the municipal system even more attractive as locations for residencies.

The overall outlook with respect to medical staffing policy is that there is potential for both reduced costs and increased quality if current arrangements are reconsidered. The HHC leadership should be in a good position to bargain for lower-cost medical care services from those institutions that are willing and able to maintain teaching affiliations and medical staff without maintaining large teaching programs.

## Notes

1. Much of the historical material in this section is adapted from Miriam Ostow, "Affiliations," in Eli Ginzberg and the Conservation of Human Resources Staff, *Urban Health Services: The Case of New York* (New York: Columbia University Press, 1971).
2. Charles Brecher, *Where Have All the Dollars Gone?* (New York: Praeger Publishers, 1974), p. 22 (Table 23).
3. The following paragraphs draw upon material in Chapter 2 of Robert Alford, *Health Care Politics* (Chicago: University of Chicago Press, 1975).
4. See *Community Health Services for New York City: Report and Staff Studies of the Commission on the Delivery of Personal Health Services* (New York: Praeger Publishers, 1969), esp. pp. 302–17.
5. See Robb K. Burlage, *New York City's Municipal Hospitals: A Policy Review* (Washington, DC: Institute for Policy Studies, 1967).
6. This discussion draws upon Charles Brecher and Miriam Ostow, "Ambulatory Care," in *Urban Health Services*; and Chapter 3 in Robert Alford, *Health Care Politics*.
7. Figures are from one-day patient censuses conducted by Blue Cross and reported in Joan Lieman, "Federal Financing and Local Control" (Ph.D. diss., Columbia University, 1977).
8. Lieman, "Federal Financing and Local Control" (Table 5.2).

9. *Health Care Needs and the New York City Health and Hospitals Corporation* (State Study Commission for New York City, April 1973), p. 175.
10. Lieman, "Federal Financing and Local Control," p. 144.
11. This discussion draws from sections on the HHC in "Mayor's Management Report" (New York City Office of Operations, annual editions for 1978–85). It should be noted that ongoing concerns involving improvements in financial performance, the opening of Woodhull Hospital, and improvement of the citywide emergency medical service are not included in the discussion because they are not illustrative of the types of programmatic concerns being discussed; however, these were major concerns and accomplishments of HHC management during this period.
12. David Axelrod, "The State Perspective," *Bulletin of the New York Academy of Medicine* 62, no. 1 (January–February 1986): 98.
13. *Report of the New York State Commission on Graduate Medical Education* (Albany: New York State Department of Health, September 1985).
14. In reviewing drafts of this analysis, HHC officials noted several aspects of the national model described in Chapter 7 that limit its ability to predict accurately the costs of individual HHC hospitals. These include the large number of alternate level of care days at HHC facilities, the inclusion of certain ambulance service costs in HHC budgets, the difficulties of case mix measures to deal with severity issues and psychiatric problems and services, and possible distortions from converting outpatient to inpatient services based on revenue weights. Despite these potential sources of inaccuracy, the findings are reasonable estimates of the extent to which HHC facilities deviate from national patterns.
15. Herbert Hyman, "Are Public Hospitals in New York City Inferior to Voluntary, Nonprofit Hospitals? A Study of JCAH Hospital Surveys," *American Journal of Public Health* 76, no. 1 (January 1981): 18–22.
16. Citizens Budget Commission, "A Report on Proposed Measures of the Volume and Quality of Services Provided by the New York City Health and Hospitals Corporation" (Report to the Josiah Macy, Jr., Foundation, November 1984).
17. Ibid.
18. Ibid.
19. See "Health Care in New York City" (Louis Harris and Associates Study no. 814009, October 1982); and Howard E. Freeman and Hye Kgung Lee, "New Yorkers' Perceptions of Their Health Care," *New York Affairs* 9, no. 2 (1985): 74–81.
20. Unpublished data from New York State Office of Health Systems Management.
21. See *Inpatient Hospital Use in New York City, 1982* (New York: United Hospital Fund, 1983).
22. In addition, a pilot program in the obstetrics department at Harlem Hospital will allow separate billing for physician services.

# ⚜ 4 ⚜

# Los Angeles County Public Hospitals

## Martha Solish

Los Angeles County operates the nation's second-largest urban public hospital system. Its six hospitals spend over $800 million annually to maintain over 3,100 beds and provide more than one million ambulatory care visits. However, the first half of the 1980s was a turbulent time for local governments in California, and the performance of Los Angeles County hospitals has been influenced by these trends as well as by more general developments in the American health care industry. This chapter begins with background material on the LA County hospitals and then describes changes in the system's performance over the 1980–84 period. The remaining four sections analyze the relationships among the policy variables — governance arrangements, financing, teaching affiliations, and market strategy — and trends in performance.

## Background

### Organizational History

Los Angeles County is governed by a board of supervisors with five members, each of whom is elected through district representation to a four-year term. The board has both legislative and executive authority over the county's departments. The board has authority to issue bonds and to levy taxes, although severe restrictions have been placed on this authority in recent years by voter referendum. A county chief administrative officer (CAO) is appointed by the board. The

## Table 4.1

## Characteristics of LA County Hospitals

| Hospital | County District | Affiliated Medical School | Staffed Beds (1984) |
|---|---|---|---|
| LAC–USC Medical Center | 3rd | University of Southern California School of Medicine | 1,432 |
| Harbor-UCLA Medical Center | 2nd | University of California at Los Angeles School of Medicine | 465 |
| King/Drew Medical Center | 2nd | Charles R. Drew Postgraduate Medical School | 440 |
| Rancho Los Amigos Medical Center | 1st | University of Southern California School of Medicine | 560 |
| Olive View Medical Center | 5th | University of California at Los Angeles School of Medicine | 122 |
| High Desert Hospital | 5th | None | 122 |

CAO's office has responsibility for the county budget and personnel systems and for other areas specified by the board.

The board meets weekly on items affecting the county's 46 departments. At these meetings, decisions are typically approved unanimously with little public discussion. Each supervisor's office has a deputy in charge of health issues, and most board actions simply ratify decisions worked out by the supervisors' staffs. Several factors explain this governance pattern. First, the vast number of areas under the board's purview limits the time available to discuss any single issue. Second, there are no standing committees of the board, and all items must be decided by the full board. Finally, the board has both legislative and administrative functions, so it must carry out its policy decisions. Members feel that public disagreement on an issue would make implementation more difficult.

There are six county hospitals, located in four of the five county supervisory districts (see Table 4.1). Three medical schools are affiliated with five of the hospitals. In 1984, fully 3,163 beds were in operation (staffed and budgeted) in the county system.

The oldest and largest hospital is the Los Angeles County–University of Southern California Medical Center (LAC-USC), which has served indigent patients in the county since 1878. It operates 1,432 beds in four separate facilities: a general hospital, a women's hospital, a pediatric pavilion, and a psychiatric hospital. It also offers 145 different training programs with 5,300 enrollees through its affiliation with the University of Southern California School of Medicine, its own school of nursing, and other affiliations.[1] LAC-USC offers a wide range of acute care services and does so in large volume. For example, in 1982 there were nearly 15,000 live births in the hospital, 10.7 percent of all births in the county.[2]

Harbor Medical Center is an acute care facility affiliated with the University of California at Los Angeles (UCLA) School of Medicine. It operates 465 beds and offers tertiary care in a number of acute care specialties. It is well known for its work in fertility and fetal surgery.

Martin Luther King, Jr.–Drew Medical Center (King/Drew) is the newest county hospital. It was built as part of the state and county response to the Watts riots of 1965, and opened in 1972. It operates 440 beds in a poor, black community that previously lacked accessible health care services. The Charles R. Drew Postgraduate Medical School, established concurrently with the hospital, provides the teaching affiliation for this institution.

Rancho Los Amigos Medical Center is a rehabilitation facility. It is affiliated with USC and operates 560 beds out of a total capacity of 969 beds. A skilled nursing program previously operated at Long Beach General Hospital (a county hospital that closed in 1983) was transferred to Rancho.

The other two county hospitals are smaller facilities. High Desert Hospital is located in a rural portion of the county 75 miles from downtown Los Angeles. It operates 122 beds and offers acute medical, surgical, and skilled nursing facilities. It has no medical training program. Olive View Medical Center occupied a temporary facility following the destruction of the hospital in a 1971 earthquake. A new 350-bed facility opened in 1987. The hospital operates general medical, surgical, pediatric, and psychiatric services and is affiliated with UCLA.

The Los Angeles County hospitals have always been governed as a unit of the county government. They depend on the county for overall administration, budgeting, policy, personnel, and long-range planning decisions. There are no independent boards overseeing the hospitals, either separately or as a group. The hospitals account for operating revenues and expenses within separate enterprise funds, but each hospital must return any surplus to the county's general fund.

Historically, county hospital administrators worked closely with the supervisor in their district. Supervisors generally served as advocates for their hospitals. Each supervisor had a high degree of autonomy regarding the use of his or her "own" hospital; one interviewee noted that each hospital used to be governed separately, "almost like a duchy."

A series of reorganizations that began in 1972 has sought to reduce the individual supervisors' autonomy and impose more professional administrative practices on the county hospital system. The Los Angeles County Department of Health Services (DHS) was formed in 1972 by merging the former departments of hospitals, public health, and comparative medical and veterinary services. (Mental health was also included initially but separated in 1978). However, the DHS retained a geographic organization, with five districts corresponding to the county board's supervisory districts.

Other factors also made a merger of the departments of public health and hospitals seem desirable at the beginning of the 1970s.[3] First, consistent with actions in some other large cities, mergers were viewed as efficiency measures. The new consolidated unit was expected to have lower overhead costs and to be more effective in collecting third-party revenues, especially for ambulatory care services often previously provided "free" at public health clinics. Second, state legislation passed in the wake of federal Medicaid legislation made a merger financially attractive to the county because state reimbursement for public health services could be applied to public health facilities. Although this favorable state legislation was repealed in 1971, the county moved ahead with merger plans in the hope of achieving efficiency gains by integrating ambulatory care services.

The county elections of 1980 brought a shift on the board of supervisors from a Democratic to a Republican majority, and this new orientation continues to the present. Major policy changes followed this shift, reflecting a new conservative majority. The new policies emphasized less spending on hospitals and a greater commitment to criminal justice and other services. Issues of access receive a lower priority, and cost containment measures such as private sector contracting and patient billing are emphasized.

To implement these policies effectively, the board reorganized the DHS in 1980. The geographic base of organization was replaced with a functional one. Four major operational units were created: public health, ambulatory care, LAC-USC Medical Center, and hospitals (which included the five other county hospitals). Each unit was administered by a deputy director who reported to the director of health services. In 1985, the organizational structure was further refined by the appointment of three assistant directors to whom the deputy directors report: one in charge of all county hospitals, one in charge of administrative and financial services, and the third in charge of all other programs.

The successive organizational changes have created a governance structure based more on functional than on geographic groupings. This increasingly functional hierarchy has been accompanied by a diminution of the hospital–district supervisor relationship and has led to greater hospital dependency on the centralized county administrative staff. However, there is still a close working relationship between each hospital administrator and the appropriate supervisor and supervisor's staff.

### Regulatory Environment

California's hospital industry is highly competitive and is characterized by decreasing inpatient utilization and a growing trend toward reduced payments by public and private insurers. In 1982, the statewide occupancy rate was 66.1 percent, compared with a national rate of 73.5 percent; in Los Angeles County the rate was an even lower 64.4 percent.[4] With 170 acute care hospitals and over 31,000 available beds, Los Angeles County is considered overbedded.

Despite the abundant bed supply, the state has not sought to use its regulating authority to curb further expansions. The certificate of need program was suspended in 1987 and the state has allowed new construction in recent years.

The state also supports one of the most expensive Medicaid programs in the nation, known as Medi-Cal. The program's eligibility rules are relatively generous, covering both those receiving public assistance and a medically needy group. The maximum income for Medi-Cal eligibility in 1987 was $1,009 monthly for a family of four. This income level slightly exceeded the federal poverty level. In 1980 Medi-Cal enrollees represented 83 percent of those below the poverty level in California, a figure well above the average for all states.[5]

In 1982, in response to severe budgetary pressures, the state enacted two fundamental reforms in Medi-Cal. First, responsibility for medical services to medically indigent adults (MIAs) was transferred from the Medi-Cal program to county governments. To help finance this care, the state provided financial assistance by providing counties approximately 70 percent of the state's previous expenditures for this group under Medi-Cal. Los Angeles, like most counties, responded to this action by limiting MIAs' eligibility to services only from county hospitals. Thus, the state's policy had the effect of substantially increasing utilization of county facilities.

The initial 70 percent payment rate may have provided financial gains to the county because the marginal cost of additional patients at county hospitals probably was less than the amount of the new state revenues. However, county officials expected that the state would redirect the payments as a percentage of costs in future years, and this did in fact happen. Thus, the financial gains to the county from the 1982 MIA transfer were relatively short-lived.

The second important feature of the 1982 reforms was a shift to a policy of selective contracting with hospitals for Medi-Cal services. Under this approach, the state negotiated a per diem rate with each hospital wanting to care for Medi-Cal patients. Beneficiaries can receive services only at the hospitals that negotiate contracts, and contracts are granted only to hospitals meeting the state's criteria, including stringent budget objectives. Initially the state planned to reduce hospital expenditures under Medi-Cal by $200 million annually through selective contracting. All LA County hospitals received contracts under the program, but several large private hospitals in the county did not. Thus, this aspect of the reforms also had the effect of channelling additional utilization to the county system.

Finally, it should be noted that the 1982 legislation also permitted private insurers in the state to engage in selective contracting. Given California's abundant bed supply, insurers have been able to obtain discounted prices from hospitals, and preferred provider organizations (PPOs) have proliferated in the state. This growing practice of selective contracting has limited hospitals' ability to finance indigent care through cost shifting.

## Trends in Performance

The performance of LA County public hospitals, particularly with respect to efficiency and access, showed significant improvement in the early 1980s. The following subsections of this chapter discuss trends in efficiency, access, and quality of care, and the remainder of the chapter links them to aspects of governance, financing, teaching arrangements, and market strategy.

### Efficiency

The LA County public hospital system began the 1980s with relatively high unit costs. From 1980 through 1982, the county's public hospitals had average daily costs and average costs per admission significantly higher than those of all relevant comparison groups (see Table 4.2). These higher costs stemmed from both relatively high staff-to-work-load ratios and relatively high salary levels. In 1982 LA County public hospitals' ratio of staff to average daily census was 5.7, well above the figures for all state and local hospitals in California (4.7) and for hospitals nationwide (3.8). In addition, average 1982 salary

## Table 4.2

## Relative Efficiency of LA County Public Hospitals, 1980–84

| | 1980 | 1981 | 1982 | 1983 | 1984 |
|---|---|---|---|---|---|
| **Operating Expenses per Adjusted Patient Day**[a] | | | | | |
| Public hospitals in LA County | $521 | $563 | $666 | $658 | $647 |
| State and local government hospitals in California | 374 | 429 | 507 | 546 | 583 |
| Community hospitals in California | 362 | 428 | 507 | 565 | 603 |
| State and local government hospitals in U.S. | 239 | 274 | 312 | 348 | 385 |
| Community hospitals in U.S. | 245 | 284 | 327 | 369 | 411 |
| **Operating Expenses per Adjusted Admission**[a] | | | | | |
| Public hospitals in LA County | $2,959 | $3,302 | $3,729 | $3,189 | $3,598 |
| State and local government hospitals in California | 2,560 | 2,939 | 3,442 | 3,688 | 3,815 |
| Community hospitals in California | 2,395 | 2,809 | 3,311 | 3,635 | 3,787 |
| State and local government hospitals in U.S. | 1,750 | 2,072 | 2,364 | 2,621 | 2,823 |
| Community hospitals in U.S. | 1,851 | 2,171 | 2,501 | 2,789 | 2,995 |
| **FTE Staff per Adjusted Average Daily Census** | | | | | |
| Public hospitals in LA County | 5.1[b] | 5.8 | 5.7 | 5.2 | 5.0 |
| State and local government hospitals in California | 4.2 | 4.2 | 4.7 | 4.2 | 5.5 |
| Community hospitals in California | 3.9 | 4.1 | 4.5 | 4.3 | 4.4 |
| State and local government hospitals in U.S. | 3.4 | 3.5 | 3.8 | 3.6 | 4.4 |
| Community hospitals in U.S. | 3.4 | 3.5 | 3.8 | 3.6 | 3.7 |

Sources: Los Angeles County DHS, annual reports and correspondence dated 28 October 1985; *Statistical Guide*, 1980–1984 editions (Chicago: American Hospital Association, 1981–1985).

[a]Adjusted inpatient services include an adjustment for outpatient service volume based on the ratio of outpatient revenue to inpatient revenue.

[b]Figure excludes King/Drew Medical Center because data are unavailable.

## Table 4.3

## Staff and Salary Levels at Urban Public Teaching Hospitals, 1982

| | LA County Hospitals | | | | | Urban Public Teaching Hospitals in Western Region | U.S. Urban Public Teaching Hospitals |
|---|---|---|---|---|---|---|---|
| | LAC-USC[a] | Harbor-UCLA | King/Drew | Rancho | High Desert | | |
| Staff per 10,000 adjusted patient days | 165.5 | 151.1 | 168.0 | 142.0 | 84.2 | 152.7 | 132.2 |
| RNs per 10,000 adjusted patient days | 25.0 | 35.5 | 19.1 | 19.8 | 7.9 | 29.2 | 26.4 |
| LPNs and VPNs per 10,000 adjusted patient days | 7.0 | 8.2 | 9.0 | 5.2 | 2.4 | 7.9 | 7.1 |
| Residents per 10,000 adjusted patient days | 14.5 | 21.3 | 23.4 | 2.4 | 0.0 | 12.1 | 9.1 |
| Physicians/dentists per 10,000 adjusted patient days | 7.0 | 9.0 | 9.3 | 5.5 | 7.5 | 2.5 | 3.0 |
| Average salary per FTE employee[b] | $19.6 | $22.8 | $20.5 | $21.0 | $21.4 | $17.4 | $16.4 |
| Average salary per FTE physician[b] | 69.4 | 61.7 | 64.3 | 66.1 | 53.6 | 94.6 | 61.3 |
| Average salary per FTE nurse[b] | 20.7 | 15.9 | 23.9 | 13.6 | 25.8 | 21.0 | 19.6 |
| Payroll expense as a percentage of total expenses | 55.6% | 61.8% | 48.8% | 52.3% | 55.3% | 51.1% | 51.0% |
| Employee benefits as a percentage of payroll expense | 24.9% | 24.0% | 25.1% | 25.3% | 24.3% | 23.1% | 19.2% |

Source: Unpublished tabulation from Urban Institute data base.

[a]General hospital only. Also, data from Olive View Medical Center are unavailable.

[b]In thousands of dollars.

## Table 4.4

## Service Volume of LA County Department of Health Services, Fiscal Years 1980–84

|  | 1980 | 1981 | 1982 | 1983 | 1984 |
|---|---|---|---|---|---|
| Admissions | 138,739 | 142,829 | 137,830 | 155,150 | 163,091 |
| Patient days | 989,342 | 984,226 | 903,429 | 976,196 | 1,003,075 |
| Average length of stay (days) | 7.1 | 6.9 | 6.6 | 6.3 | 6.2 |
| Bed complement | 3,191 | 3,195 | 3,043 | 2,921 | 3,163 |
| Occupancy rate | 84.9% | 84.4% | 81.3% | 91.6% | 86.9% |
| Total ambulatory care visits | 1,168,395 | 1,049,593 | 887,832 | 938,928 | 1,059,720 |
|    Outpatient department visits | 816,481 | 723,806 | 633,163 | 676,179 | 781,590 |
|    Emergency room visits | 351,914 | 325,787 | 242,859 | 262,758 | 278,136 |
| Full-time-equivalent employees | NA | 20,149 | 17,475 | 17,293 | 17,201 |
| Operating expenses (in thousands of dollars) | $649,358 | $708,432 | $741,593 | $796,698 | $816,432 |

Source: Los Angeles County DHS correspondence dated 28 October 1985.

NA: Not available.

levels at LA County hospitals ranged from $19,600 to $22,800, compared to a regional average of $17,400 and a national average of $16,400 (see Table 4.3).

However, beginning in 1982 the LA County hospital system made some significant gains in relative efficiency. Between 1982 and 1984, average costs per day and per admission actually fell by 2.8 percent and 3.5 percent, respectively. In contrast, the corresponding national averages jumped 25.7 percent and 19.8 percent. While LA County hospitals' per diem costs were still above those at other hospitals in 1984, the gap was significantly narrowed. Moreover, costs per adjusted admission at LA County hospitals actually fell below those at other California hospitals in 1983 and 1984.

The significant gains in relative efficiency resulted from staff reductions initiated in 1982 combined with increases in service volume beginning in 1983. Between 1982 and 1983 the DHS reduced its hospital staff over 13 percent, from 20,149 to 17,475. In 1983 and 1984, staff declines continued to 17,293 and 17,201, respectively. At the same time, the hospital's service volume increased (see Table 4.4). Between 1982 and 1984, admissions rose over 18 percent, days over 11 percent, and ambulatory care visits over 19 percent. In the same period, total operating costs increased only 10 percent. Thus, the most significant efficiency improvements were related to increases in patient volume

Table 4.5

## Primary Payer for Inpatient Admissions at
## LA County Hospitals, Fiscal Years 1982-85
## (percentage distribution)

|  | 1982 | 1983 | 1984 | 1985[a] |
|---|---|---|---|---|
| Medi-Cal[b] | 56.9% | 49.3% | 42.4% | 40.8% |
| Self-pay[b] | 24.1 | 31.7 | 39.7 | 42.6 |
| Indigent subtotal | 81.0 | 81.0 | 82.1 | 83.4 |
| Medicare | 7.4 | 7.2 | 6.3 | 5.5 |
| Private insurance | 6.9 | 5.7 | 5.2 | 5.2 |
| Short-Doyle[c] | 1.7 | 3.7 | 4.0 | 3.5 |
| Other | 3.0 | 2.4 | 2.5 | 2.5 |
| Total | 100.0% | 100.0% | 100.0% | 100.0% |

Source: Correspondence from Los Angeles County DHS dated 1 March 1985.

Note: Primary payer is determined at admission and after 30 days of hospitalization.

[a]Based on year-to-date information through December 1984.

[b]In 1982 Medi-Cal category includes MIAs; in 1983-85 MIAs are included in self-pay category.

[c]Refers to mental health patients financed 90 percent by state funds and 10 percent by county funds.

that occurred after the Medi-Cal reforms. However, as will be discussed below, the efficiency gains suggested by these measures may not adequately reflect the changes in quality of care and access to care that accompanied the increases in service volume.

### Access

State law and county DHS policies specify that the primary purpose of the county hospitals is to serve "all indigent persons who are resident" in the county. The county hospitals also serve a large number of undocumented immigrants. Services to nonindigent individuals are to be provided only when capacity is available.

In light of this mission, it is not surprising that the vast majority of DHS facility patients are indigent. From 1982 through 1985 at least 81 percent of all admissions to county hospitals were indigents (see Table 4.5). Privately insured patients accounted for only between 5 and 7 percent of admissions.

Given the consistent, dominant role of indigents among DHS patients, trends in total services can be equated with trends in services to this group. The figures in Table 4.4 reveal contrasting developments in the 1980-82 and the 1982-84 periods. In the first two years, inpatient services remained relatively stable while ambulatory care was reduced substantially. Emergency room visits declined 31 percent and other outpatient visits dropped over 22 percent. In the 1982–84 period all types of service were markedly expanded; admissions rose 18 percent and ambulatory care visits rose 19 percent. The connections between these abrupt shifts in utilization and the policy variables considered in this study are discussed in the sections that follow.

## Quality

In California, accreditation surveys are performed by the Joint Commission on Accreditation of Healthcare Organizations in collaboration with the California Medical Association (CMA) and the State Department of Health Services. These surveys may result in accreditation for up to three years, contingent on correction of specifically identified deficiencies.

In their most recent surveys, all of the LA County hospitals obtained three-year accreditation, and all deficiencies cited were corrected. One of the hospitals, Harbor-UCLA, had no deficiencies in its latest survey. LAC-USC had several deficiencies related to building and safety codes but none relating to clinical care.

Despite the generally favorable survey findings, there have been recurring concerns over the quality of clinical care in parts of the county system. The Joint Commission survey and reports in the media questioned the quality of surgical care delivered at King/Drew. The survey indicated that thorough physical examinations were not completed prior to surgery. The CMA reviews noted a high percentage of normal appendices removed at Olive View and of complications from invasive radiological procedures at LAC-USC. The special care unit at High Desert Hospital had not been licensed before the latest survey (1985), although this was later remedied. Other deficiencies related to inadequate equipment; for example, inadequate resuscitation equipment was cited in the delivery room at LAC-USC. Insufficient staffing caused nuclear medicine tests to be backlogged up to three days at LAC-USC, and nurses frequently worked double shifts at King/Drew.

However, most of the problems cited in the Joint Commission and CMA surveys related to physical plant problems, which can be traced to inadequate capital investment. The main hospital at LAC-USC has not been substantially renovated since 1933, and many building and safety deficiencies were noted in its Joint Commission report. Other deficiencies related to the lack of adequate housekeeping and facility maintenance. Overall, the average age of plant in the county system was 14 years in 1982, compared to a national average of 6.3 years.[6]

Another frequently used indicator of quality of care is the percentage of foreign medical graduates (FMGs) among first-year residents at a hospital. The three LA County hospitals for which these data were available vary widely on this measure. The national average is 15.4 percent. At King/Drew, fully 62 percent of first-year residents were FMGs in 1983–84, compared with only 7 percent at both Harbor-UCLA and LAC-USC.[7] The high percentage of FMGs at King/Drew may indicate a lower quality of care, but it may also reflect that hospital's reputation for outstanding tropical medicine training. The low percentage of FMGs at the other two major medical centers supports a Joint Commission finding of high quality clinical care. While lacking the physical attractiveness of many hospitals, the LA County facilities seem to provide an adequate quality of clinical care, even outstanding in some areas.

Numerous newspaper articles and studies have found that termination of Medi-Cal benefits for MIA patients resulted in increased waiting times and delayed treatment.[8] These findings suggest that the quality of care received by some patients declined because the increased demand for services after MIA transfer exceeded the county's additional health care resources. Many have argued that the efficiency gains cited earlier (measured by expenses incurred per adjusted admission) were achieved at the expense of quality of care, although the data are not conclusive on this point.

## Governance

### Current Arrangements

LA County's hospitals have always been operated directly as a unit of local government under the board of supervisors. However, within this general system there have been two important changes in recent years. First, internal reorganizations have sought to tighten the control of professional administrators in the central office over hospital management, with consequent reductions in direct links between hospital administrators and the supervisor in each hospital's district. Second, the party composition, and hence philosophical orientation, of the board of supervisors has changed. Each of these changes has implications for the pattern of governance and for the hospital system's performance.

Although becoming less important, the relationship between the individual supervisors' offices and the individual hospital administrators is generally characterized by both sides as positive. Supervisors pay close attention to health care issues because DHS is the single largest department in the county budget and because hospitals are highly visible facilities with strong community support. The supervisors' deputies in charge of health care issues meet weekly with the director of DHS to discuss departmental issues.

The close involvement of supervisors and their deputies in health care issues is generally helpful to hospital administrators. It provides them with direct access to the top county decision makers, in place of routing communications through each hospital's assistant director at DHS and the county administrative officer as specified in DHS guidelines. However, senior DHS staff feel that these alternative communication paths weaken their authority and fragment control over the hospitals.

Hospital administrators generally are critical of the central county offices and their departmental headquarters. The administrators resent the high degree of centralization, which they feel prevents innovative decision making. They do not perceive civil service regulations as allowing for decentralized personnel decisions.

The election of a conservative Republican majority to the board of supervisors in 1980 was accompanied by a major change in board philosophy, including a greater emphasis on cost containment. The new board considered and adopted several distinct strategies to reduce hospital costs. The following sections discuss these strategies and the controversy generated by them.

## Implications of Governance Policies

The most striking effect of the changed board policies was to increase efficiency. The board conveyed to service managers a clear sense of the importance of reducing unit costs, and rewarded and punished managers based on their results. A variety of productivity improvement programs were developed, and somewhat greater flexibility within the civil service system was achieved.

The most visible of the board's efforts is a comprehensive campaign to increase contracting with the private sector. Board policy is that such contracts will be employed "when economy or efficiency is promoted and such contracting is appropriate to the service."[9] Most new contracts have been for support services, including food preparation, laundry, and custodial services. In addition, in 1985 a contract was awarded for financial management services at King/Drew, and contracting for clinical services (physical therapy and laboratory services) was underway. By the end of 1984, a total of 21 contracts had been signed, achieving an estimated annual savings of $4.8 million.[10]

The board of supervisors has also considered the most extreme version of contracting out: the sale of a public hospital. In 1982 a blue-ribbon committee was appointed to consider the sale of Rancho Los Amigos to National Medical Enterprises. Precedent had been set in California by the sale of county hospitals in Sacramento, San Diego, and Orange Counties. The unions, whose goal was to retain county jobs for their largely minority membership, strongly opposed the plan. The board eventually rejected the sale. Some observers believe that formal consideration was given to the idea only as an implicit threat to encourage other efficiency measures at the hospital.

## Financing

During the 1980–84 period the financing of the LA County hospitals was changed in two important ways. First, subsidies from the county were reduced because Proposition 13, a statewide tax limitation measure, reduced resources available to the county. Second, the changes in the state Medicaid program reduced resources from that program, although they provided new state revenues for an enlarged number of medically indigent patients. Both changes had significant implications for the county hospital system's performance.

### Reductions in County Support

Historically, the Los Angeles County hospitals received a substantial subsidy from the county. The county's relatively sound financial condition enabled it to provide what was widely considered to be generous funding levels to the Department of Health Services, its largest agency. In the 1970s, the county subsidy accounted for roughly 50 percent of the hospitals' revenues; receipts from private insurers never accounted for more than 10 percent.[11]

The Medi-Cal Reform Act of 1971 was a precursor of change in this situation. This law virtually eliminated the state subsidy to the counties for public hospitals. In addition, it put upon the counties the burden of paying for part of the state's share of total Medi-Cal expenses. This legislation came at the time of the formation of the Los Angeles County Department of Health Services. Since the decision to form DHS assumed the continuation of the state contribution to public hospitals, the 1971 Act was a serious constraint on public hospitals' financing.

To make up for lost state revenues, the counties raised local taxes. As a result, health care expenditures increased from 30 percent of

## Table 4.6
## Financing of LA County Hospitals,
## Fiscal Years 1980–84
## (dollars in millions)

|  | 1980 | 1981 | 1982 | 1983 | 1984 |
|---|---|---|---|---|---|
| Medi-Cal | $199.4 | $216.0 | $304.9 | $228.5 | $237.8 |
| MIA | — | — | — | 108.4 | 162.9 |
| Medi-Cal and MIA subtotal | 199.4 | 216.0 | 304.9 | 336.9 | 400.7 |
| | | | | | |
| Medicare | 72.3 | 65.4 | 67.3 | 56.1 | 57.3 |
| Other insurance | 32.6 | 41.6 | 45.3 | 57.7 | 48.3 |
| Self-pay | 14.8 | 16.2 | 13.4 | 11.6 | 25.3 |
| Other | 69.6 | 77.0 | 67.3 | 66.7 | 71.8 |
| | | | | | |
| Net operating revenues | 388.6 | 416.3 | 498.2 | 529.0 | 603.5 |
| County subsidy | 235.6 | 257.8 | 251.8 | 220.9 | 221.6 |
| Total revenues | $624.2 | $674.1 | $750.0 | $749.9 | $825.1 |

Sources: Total operating revenues and county subsidy are based on accrued figures reported in the Los Angeles County Comprehensive Annual Financial Report for fiscal years 1980 through 1984. The amounts for each type of operating revenue are author's estimates based on an unpublished percentage distribution of cash receipts supplied by the Department of Health Services.

California counties' property tax revenues in 1966–67 to 36 percent in 1973–74.[12] Eventually, in 1978, the voters expressed their unwillingness to pay for continually rising local government expenditures, with the passage of Proposition 13. This state measure limited the size of local property tax revenues, forcing reductions in such taxes for LA and other counties. Although additional state aid helped offset some of the reduced property tax revenues, the net effect was still severe revenue constraints for the county.

With revenues limited, the county concentrated on expenditure controls. Between 1980 and 1984, the county subsidy declined from 38 percent to 27 percent of DHS hospitals' net revenues (see Table 4.6). The size of the county subsidy was unstable in this period, varying from $221 million to $258 million between 1980 and 1984 without a direct relationship to the hospital system's operating loss.

As a result of the funding restrictions caused by Proposition 13, LA County initiated copayments for health services at its hospitals. Objections to these fees by community groups resulted in the ability-to-pay (ATP) plan in September 1979. This plan required fees based on a sliding scale linked to patients' income as determined through financial screening conducted by county employees. Patients had seven days to apply for Medi-Cal or for the ATP program before they became liable for the entire fee for the visit. If the financial screening under ATP determined that the patient's income was less than $248 per month, the patient's liability would be reduced to zero. In 1981, an initial deposit of $30 was imposed at hospital clinics for all nonemergent visits. This made the ATP plan even more important for indigent patients, particularly those requiring prenatal care.

From its beginning, the ATP program was inadequately staffed. In addition, patients complained they were not aware of its existence. Some patients apparently thought that cash payments were required of everyone and left without treatment.[13] Signs placed in LAC-USC stating, "Health care is not free! Everyone must pay!" furthered this perception.[14]

To reduce the cost of the screening and make the process more equitable, a revised ATP plan (ATP-R) was adopted in March 1983. Under ATP-R, patients can declare indigency and pay $30 within seven days as an alternative to undergoing the more extensive financial screening.

The ATP plan restricted access to health care for many patients and reduced utilization of county facilities. A study of eight county health centers showed a significant drop in prenatal visits after fees were imposed.[15] A survey of county hospital patients who had received no prenatal care showed that the share who identified financial problems as the reason for not receiving care jumped from 33 percent in 1978 to 70 percent in 1982.[16] Furthermore, between 1980 and 1982, ambulatory care visits to the county hospitals decreased by 24 percent (see Table 4.4). In sum, the reduced county support led to measures that reduced access to care for the indigent.

In addition to the ATP plan, the county responded to post–Proposition 13 financial constraints by seeking to increase state revenues from the Medi-Cal program. In 1980, a new financial data acquisition system, staffed by about 200 new employees, was acquired to enhance the hospitals' ability to collect financial information from patients and encourage them to apply for Medi-Cal. One administrator reported that fully 80 percent of the Medi-Cal patients in his hospital are enrolled while at the hospital. A fivefold increase in Medi-Cal applications by undocumented immigrants was observed as a result of these efforts.[17] In fact, between 1980 and 1982 Medi-Cal revenues jumped an estimated 53 percent as a result of the increased billing efforts and the rate increases.

However, the Medi-Cal enrollment initiatives were viewed with suspicion by some undocumented immigrants and discouraged some from seeking care. Thus, this revenue enhancement program may have had the double effect of increasing Medi-Cal revenues but reducing the total number of undocumented immigrants seeking care. On the other hand, these funds permit the hospitals' budget to grow despite the constraints on the county subsidy.

Despite these Medi-Cal revenue enhancements, service reductions did occur. In fiscal year 1982, pharmacy services were cut at the four largest hospitals, and eight health centers were closed.[18] These and other measures were necessary to keep expenditure increases in line with available revenues.

Finally, Proposition 13 led the county to be very cautious about capital investments for the public hospitals. Because of the property tax limits, the county was unable to issue new general obligation bonds, and therefore has limited access to new capital. Consequently, the county hospitals have had virtually no new capital investments. An estimated $660 million is needed for capital improvements, over $300 million alone for LAC-USC.[19] As one DHS administrator stated, "the county needs a viable plan for capital financing."

## Medi-Cal Reforms

In response to the rapid increases in Medi-Cal spending, the state in 1982 enacted the significant program changes described earlier. From the vantage point of LA County hospitals the most important change was the shift from Medi-Cal coverage to county responsibility for MIAs.

There are an estimated 45,000 MIAs in Los Angeles County. Before the 1982 reforms, this group received most of its care at private hospitals; an estimated 55 percent of MIA admissions and 71 percent of MIA ambulatory visits were to noncounty facilities in 1981.[20] Under the new program, the private hospitals would not be paid by Medi-Cal for this care. Either the patients would have to shift to the county hospitals, or the private hospitals would have to increase their charity care.

Most of the hospital care for MIAs in Los Angeles was shifted to the county hospitals. In fiscal year 1983, admissions were up 12.6 percent over fiscal year 1982, patient days were up 8 percent, outpatient department volume increased 6.8 percent, and the occupancy rate at the hospitals reached its highest level ever at 91.6 percent (see Table 4.4).

Service demand increased even further in fiscal year 1984, severely straining the county hospitals' capacity in some specialties. In obstetrics, it became necessary to establish overflow contracts with private hospitals to handle the increased volume. Average waits for appointments in county ambulatory care centers increased from two weeks to six weeks.[21] Self-pay and MIA patients increased to nearly 40 percent of total admissions (see Table 4.5).

The increased volume caused some access difficulties for patients. Delays of up to four months for appointments to some specialized services were reported, with consequent greater severity of illness for those treated. Medically indigent patients also faced increased travel times, which may have limited their access to care. The combined effect of treatment delays and increased travel time on the health status of MIA patients was studied one year after the transfer. Researchers found differences in health status between a group of MIA patients and a matched control group and linked the differences to the lack of available health services for the MIA patients.[22]

On the other hand, the MIA transfer was accompanied by measures intended to reduce financial obstacles to care for the poor, including undocumented immigrants. The county was prohibited from requiring an initial deposit before providing care, because the state MIA legislation mandated that no one be denied care because of a payment requirement. This would seem to allow for enhanced access to care; nevertheless, the ATP program discussed above continued to function, and because of this program patients may not have requested care. In addition, there are reports that the prohibition of prepayment requirements was only sporadically enforced.[23]

The Medi-Cal reforms did result in short-run revenue increases and gains in efficiency. In both 1983 and 1984 the additional revenues from the MIA program more than offset the losses from Medi-Cal; by 1984 the combined total of Medi-Cal and MIA revenues was nearly $401 million, 31 percent above the comparable 1982 figure. However, some of these gains were used to justify subsequent reduced county subsidies, so total revenues did not continue to grow as rapidly.

The increases in volume and the relatively modest growth in total expenditures led to significant gains in efficiency. As noted earlier, average costs per admission fell between 1982 and 1984, and the number of staff per average daily census fell from 5.7 to 5.0 (see Table 4.2). The volume increases related to the MIA transfer help explain much of this improved performance.

## Teaching Affiliations

### Current Arrangements

The county hospitals have strong teaching affiliations. The facilities are staffed exclusively by medical school faculty and residents;

there are no private practitioners with admitting privileges. Further, each hospital is affiliated with only one medical school. (Harbor has an additional affiliation with the University of California at Riverside, for undergraduate medical education only, and these medical students are supervised by UCLA physicians.) These factors contribute to a strong dependency of the hospitals on the medical schools. The teaching programs were unanimously considered by those interviewed to be critical to staff recruitment; it was generally believed that it would be nearly impossible to obtain adequate and qualified staff without the affiliations.

The medical schools also seem to place a high priority on their county hospital affiliations, although the degree of their commitment varies. Both the UCLA and the University of Southern California (USC) medical schools are affiliated with other hospitals, but the county hospitals represent both a large number of patients providing teaching material unmatched elsewhere and a collaborative decision-making relationship. Drew Medical School is affiliated only with the county, and thus it is very dependent on this affiliation. The general picture is one of a strong level of commitment on both sides of the affiliation relationship.

Medical school faculty and the county are linked administratively through joint appointments; most key medical positions in the hospitals (including medical director and service chief) are held by physicians who also chair departments at their respective medical schools. This structure allows for policies in the two institutions to be aligned. In addition, the deans of the medical schools collaborate with hospital administrators on major decisions. The DHS medical director's office establishes policy relative to medical issues that affect all the hospitals, including emergency medical services, quality assurance, malpractice, and Joint Commission accreditation. Thus, most major medical decisions affecting the hospitals are made by physicians with dual appointments, in collaboration with county hospital administrators.

The clinical faculty and house staff are salaried by the county. As civil service employees their salaries are limited, but the county supplements these amounts with clinical teaching support funds paid in a lump sum to each medical school. The medical schools distribute these funds based on payment levels they establish. The county contracts for teaching support provide for an annual county obligation ranging in 1985 from $3.7 million at Drew to $11.5 million at USC.[24]

Despite these commonalities, the unique history and approach of each medical school causes each affiliation to differ. The character of each of these relationships warrants separate discussion.

**University of Southern California.** USC has the oldest and largest affiliation with the county system. Its ties with LAC-USC date from 1885, and it provides over 900 house staff in 21 specialties at that hospital alone. Since 1969, USC has also been affiliated with Rancho Los Amigos, where 25 residents in rehabilitation medicine are trained. Medical school officials are proud of their comprehensive residency programs, which have trained 19 percent of all physicians practicing in the state.[25] For the last 20 years, USC has been the only medical school affiliated with LAC-USC.

The relationship with LAC-USC is described as collaborative but as increasingly "cautious" in recent years. Two factors underlie this tension. First, recent county budget cuts have stymied the development of new programs sought by USC. Notably, a cancer hospital planned as a joint effort between the county and USC was cancelled by the county for budget reasons; USC then constructed its own cancer center on the medical school campus. Second, USC staff must share control over hospital decision making with county administrators and sometimes find this frustrating.

In part because of these tensions, USC decided in collaboration with National Medical Enterprises (NME) to build a private hospital across the street from LAC-USC. The medical school is building a 275- to 300-bed hospital that will be a tertiary care referral center for the NME chain.[26] This is the first instance nationwide of a for-profit company building, owning, and managing a teaching hospital. The company will be entitled to any profits from the hospital exclusive of physicians' fees. The impetus for this is that USC wanted its own hospital which it could "control" and that the new hospital would help increase physicians' supplemental incomes from private patients. The prospect of the new hospital has given USC physicians a reputation as the most entrepreneurial of the three medical schools' staffs.

The potential effects of this new hospital on the county are mixed. The new hospital could draw privately insured patients away from LAC-USC, but LAC-USC treats few such patients (about 5 percent of its total admissions). The new hospital could increase physicians' commitment to LAC-USC because they would no longer have to travel around Los Angeles to their various affiliated hospitals — they would be directly across the street.

**University of California at Los Angeles.** UCLA affiliated with the county system in the 1950s. It chose to affiliate with two county hospitals located at some distance from central Los Angeles and each other: Harbor General Hospital and Olive View Medical Center. Harbor also has its own freestanding program providing some clinical training for undergraduate medical students at the University of California at Riverside.

UCLA's affiliations are viewed positively by both the hospitals and the medical school. This is due largely to a high degree of consonance in overall approach and mission, especially in the case of Harbor. Harbor's strong tertiary care focus and its efforts to provide an academic medical center atmosphere are consistent with the medical school's interests. Harbor's Research and Education Institute (established to administer grants) and its freestanding medical education program led one UCLA representative to state that Harbor is "an arm of our teaching program." The dean's office occupies a more powerful position at UCLA than at USC; thus, medical needs are more likely to be taken into account in planning at Harbor than at LAC-USC. Plans for the redevelopment of Olive View Medical Center also are reported to include more involvement in teaching than previously, although a certain amount of conflict is expected on this subject.

**Drew Postgraduate Medical School.** Drew was created to help meet the staffing needs of the new Martin Luther King Hospital and to provide graduate training for black physicians, who tended to encounter discrimination in community hospitals. It was originally established as a graduate medical school only. In 1978, Drew entered into an agreement with UCLA to form a joint undergraduate medical program. Thus, Drew's accreditation is contingent on its continued affiliation with UCLA.

Drew's limited status and its dependency both on UCLA and on the county have contributed to a stormy relationship with the King/Drew Medical Center. Drew officials feel that the hospital managers do not involve physicians in decision making and do not accord enough importance to education and research; county administrators feel that Drew faculty are disdainful of community physicians. Recent attempts have been made to increase the involvement of the deans at the hospital. Despite their conflicts, the similarity in mission between the hospital and the medical school is striking: both are concerned with providing basic health services focusing on primary care to poor minority populations. The King/Drew affiliation seems to be the most troubled of the three, but each of the two institutions is attempting to accommodate the other.

## Implications of Teaching Affiliations

The principal implication of the affiliation relationships is conflict over county efforts to contain costs. This is evident in unsuccessful efforts to curb duplication of services among the hospitals and in somewhat more successful efforts by the county to reduce unit costs.

While the county's goal is to deliver quality patient care as economically as possible, the medical schools are interested primarily in research and teaching. The patient care goal is best met by concentrating specialized and expensive services, such as cardiac surgery, in one facility. But each medical school prefers to have its own specialized service programs. As a result, for example, there are open-heart surgery facilities at LAC-USC, Harbor-UCLA, and King/Drew. Duplication of services occurs in other areas as well; there are, for instance, two renal transplant services in the county system (see Table 4.7). As noted by one county hospital administrator, "Academic physicians don't have a sense for cost containment."

The affiliated medical staffs have also been a source of opposition to the county's efforts to lower its subsidy and total hospital expenditures. Medical school representatives complain that the county has been unable to maintain equipment and staffing at a level adequate for accessible and high quality care, and that the county has been unable to undertake innovative measures (such as the cancer hospital discussed above) that would improve the hospitals' service mix and community standing.

## Market Strategy

California's Welfare and Institutions Code places responsibility for indigent health care on the counties. This legislation provides for the counties to "relieve and support" all "lawful residents" in need of care who are not financially supported by other means.[27] The phrase "relieve and support" is vague, but Los Angeles County has interpreted it broadly. The county has provided care to anyone in need, including large numbers of undocumented immigrants. It has been argued that undocumented immigrants should be included in the definition of lawful resident and therefore must be part of the population included in the mandate. It is contended that the term "lawful resident" was originally intended to specify the county of residence, not whether the person was documented or not. Regardless of the outcome of the legal debate, the question of how to provide and finance the health care

## Table 4.7
### Selected Services Offered at LA County Hospitals, 1983

| | LAC-USC | Harbor-UCLA | King/Drew | OVMC | RLA | High Desert |
|---|---|---|---|---|---|---|
| Cardiac care unit | X | X | X | | | |
| Intensive care unit | X | X | X | X | X | |
| Open-heart surgery | X | X | X | | | |
| Ultrasound | X | X | X | X | X | X |
| Radiation therapy | X | X | | | | |
| Therapeutic radioisotope therapy | X | X | | X | | |
| Organ transplant | X | X | X | | | |
| Skilled nursing unit | | | | | | X |
| Burn care | X | | | | | |
| Organized OPD | X | X | X | X | X | X |
| Emergency room | X | X | X | X | | |
| Obstetrics | X | X | X | | | X |
| CT scanner | X | X | X | | X | |
| Cardiac catheterization | X | X | X | X | | |
| Neonatal intensive care | X | X | X | | | |
| Renal transplant | X | X | | | | |

Source: *1984 Guide to the Health Care Field* (Chicago: American Hospital Association, 1985).

needed by undocumented aliens is a controversial aspect of county health care services.

The county's mission excludes certain services and populations. DHS policies are that the indigent population is the "primary target of personal health services" and that services are provided to others only to increase the revenues available to serve the population specified in the legal mandate.[28] In the past, LAC-USC had a policy of excluding privately insured patients to reduce the county work load. Currently, there is debate over whether county hospitals should be allowed to offer elective services to privately insured patients.

DHS policies also state that professional education programs are "in the interest of assuring quality of service and continued supply of quality staff."[29] In other words, these programs are not ends in themselves but means to aid the mission of indigent care. Despite the fact that several county facilities are among the most prestigious education and research sites in the country, county officials stress that the county does not fund research and that medical school affiliations are the only way to obtain needed staff.

The payer mix at county hospitals reflects the mission of the hospitals as providers of last resort. In 1984, county hospital admissions were almost 40 percent self-pay and MIA patients, over 42 percent Medi-Cal, and only 5 percent privately insured (these are mostly trauma patients) (see Table 4.5). Given the large concentration of indigent patients, it is not surprising that the county system is the area's major source of care for the indigent. While representing only 13 percent of all general acute care days, the county hospitals accounted for nearly half of all bad debt and charity care and over one-third of all Medi-Cal payments in the county.[30] In addition, the high percentage of admissions originating in the emergency room—fully 92 percent at LAC-USC—attests to the hospitals' role as providers of indigent and emergency care.[31]

The service mix also reflects the hospitals' role. The county hospitals provided 21 percent of all neonatal intensive care days in the county, nearly 19 percent of all pediatric patient days, and nearly 18 percent of all emergency visits (see Table 4.8). These are services that generally reach a large number of indigent patients.

In keeping with their general mission, the county hospitals' efforts to expand their markets have generally been limited to capturing a larger share of the Medi-Cal population. The county began in 1985 to market a primary care HMO to Medi-Cal patients at King/Drew and LAC-USC. Because the plan requires enrollees to give up their Medi-Cal cards and receive all their care from county facilities, enrollment has been low. The county is trying to attract patients to the HMO

## Table 4.8

## LA County Hospitals'
## Market Share of Patient Days, 1982

| Service | LA County Hospitals Days/Visits | Total Days/Visits | LA County Hospitals' Share of Total |
|---|---|---|---|
| General acute care | 865,864 | 6,520,638 | 13.3% |
| Medical-surgical | 413,194 | 5,044,015 | 8.2 |
| Intensive care* | 64,069 | 625,694 | 10.2 |
| Pediatric | 51,970 | 276,634 | 18.8 |
| Perinatal | 74,560 | 434,695 | 17.2 |
| Intensive care newborn nursery | 26,635 | 126,436 | 21.1 |
| Burn center | 5,283 | 13,164 | 40.1 |
| Acute psychiatric | 99,013 | 719,813 | 13.8 |
| Acute rehabilitation | 105,870 | 243,154 | 43.5 |
| Live births | 24,193 | 139,930 | 17.3 |
| Emergency visits | 381,256 | 2,143,687 | 17.8 |

Source: "1984 Area Health Services and Facilities Plan" (Office of Statewide Health Planning and Development, June 1984).

*Includes ICU, CCU, and acute respiratory care.

concept through a "visibility program," in which an audiovisual presentation is made to newly eligible Medi-Cal recipients. Another effort to market services to Medi-Cal patients is a state-initiated pilot project called Expanded Choice, under which the county will offer a capitation program in competition with other providers. These efforts have proceeded cautiously to avoid the adverse reactions of private hospitals that are also seeking Medi-Cal patients.

In 1984, the county adopted a somewhat more competitive market orientation. The DHS instituted a formal planning process. (The former director of DHS had considered long-range planning to be a useless activity since the board of supervisors held all the major decision-making power.) Seven priority areas for growth were identified, and external consultants were hired to help design the long-range planning process. Other marketing efforts include a new patient services improvement project, designed partly to attract paying patients, and identification of desirable aesthetic improvements.

Rancho Los Amigos is considered to be best able to market its services to private patients because it has few nearby competitors and a relatively large base (about 12 percent) of privately insured patients. The hospital is renovating a ward for private patients and has a PPO contract with Blue Cross. Similarly, High Desert Hospital has built a new rehabilitation ward, to attract privately insured patients.

However, compared with the efforts made in the private sector, this shift toward a competitive focus is barely perceptible. The county has continued to be cautious in its marketing efforts and mindful of its legal mandate to serve the indigent. The county has been embroiled in lawsuits over the question of whether it is legally enjoined from providing services to anyone beyond the mandated population. Physicians and private hospitals have also brought the issue to light in public discussions. Finally, the county is widely conceded to have little chance of significantly increasing its private patient share. One important purpose behind its marketing efforts is to show its indispensability in the health care system and the need for continued governmental support.

## *Summary*

The LA County public hospital system is operated as a unit of local government, depends heavily on the county for operating subsidies, has strong teaching affiliations, and has remained primarily a provider of last resort for the indigent. During the early 1980s the major changes in this pattern of operation related to financing arrangements. The county sought to reduce its subsidies, and the state altered its Medicaid program in ways that directed additional patients and revenues to the county system. Thus, the principal lessons from the LA experience relate to the effect of financing changes on hospital performance.

The first important financial alteration was post–Proposition 13 reductions in support from the county. The hospitals' responses to this were primarily to reduce access and initiate measures to improve efficiency. They reduced access through the imposition of copayment requirements and financial screening for sliding-scale fee systems. In addition, they reduced staff and closed some clinics. These measures reduced care to the indigent, but had little effect on hospital efficiency. Because utilization declined as rapidly or more rapidly than did revenues or staff, the LA County hospitals continued to operate with relatively high unit costs despite resource constraints.

In contrast, the Medi-Cal changes resulted in both a larger volume of care to the indigent at LA County hospitals and greater efficiency at these facilities. The transfer of responsibility for MIAs from Medi-Cal to the county facilities limited the freedom of some indigent residents to select their provider and probably reduced their overall utilization of care. But these changes also increased the role of county hospitals in caring for the indigent and raised the volume of care the county system provided.

Since the revenues under the program did not rise as rapidly as did utilization (in part because the county continued to limit its subsidy), the hospital managers had to respond with some combination of improved efficiency and reduced quality of care. There is clear evidence that unit costs declined, suggesting some efficiency gains, but the implications for quality of care are harder to isolate. Presumably the reduction in resources per unit of service lowered quality in some way, but the stress on the hospitals probably also enhanced efficiency. Accessibility of care also suffered in the sense that some patients faced additional travel and waiting times and possible financial obstacles in the form of copayment requirements.

In contrast to the rapidly changing financing pattern, the LA county hospitals' teaching programs and market strategy have changed little and appear likely to remain stable. The close ties with area medical schools help ensure adequate medical staff, and the affiliations seem to contribute positively to quality of care. However, these teaching activities are related to the hospitals' relatively high unit costs. The hospitals' mandate requires that they focus almost exclusively on care to the indigent rather than on competing for private patients. While the hospitals' managers have developed some initiatives to market their services to Medi-Cal patients who use private hospitals, the hospitals generally remain noncompetitive with respect to privately insured patients. This situation is not likely to change, given the county hospitals' poor physical plant and image as a last-resort provider and medical staff's preference for admitting their private patients to other facilities.

## Notes

1. Data supplied by LAC-USC Medical Center.
2. Office of Statewide Health Planning and Development, "1984 Area Health Survey and Facilities Plan" (State of California, June 1984), Appendix A.
3. For additional background on the merger, see William Shonick, "Mergers of Public Health Departments with Public Hospitals in Urban Areas: Findings of 12 Field Studies," *Medical Care*, supplement (August 1980).
4. "Disclosure Reports for Fiscal Year 1982" (California Health Facilities Commission, 1984).
5. D. Sawyer, M. Ruther, A. Pagan-Berlucchi, and D. Muse, *The Mental Retardation and Medicaid Data Book, 1983* (Baltimore: U.S. Health Care Financing Administration, December 1983), pp. 91–93.

6. Figures are unpublished data from the Urban Institute, based on COTH Urban Public Hospitals Database, 1982.

7. *1984 Directory of the Council on Teaching Hospitals* (Washington, DC: Council on Teaching Hospitals, 1985).

8. N. Lurie et al., "Termination from Medi-Cal: Does It Affect Health?" *New England Journal of Medicine* 311 (30 August 1984): 480–84; and A. Scott, "County Funding Plan: Health Budget Holds Line," *Los Angeles Times*, 3 May 1983.

9. "Strategic Plan" (Los Angeles County Department of Health Services, September 1984), p. 2 (Exhibit 2).

10. "DHS, Productivity Index: Second Quarter FY 1984–85" (Correspondence from Fran Dowling to Robert Gates, February 1985), Attachment 2.

11. Estimates based on interviews with county hospital staff.

12. E. Richard Brown, "Public Hospitals on the Brink: Their Problems and Their Options, *Journal of Health Politics, Policy and Law* 7 (Winter 1983): 927–44.

13. D. Townsend, "Rising Prenatal Care Needs Noted: Policy Change May Allow More Women to Get Assistance," *Los Angeles Times*, 1 December 1982.

14. H. Nelson, "Fee Emphasis Deters Poor's Health Care, Panel Hears," *Los Angeles Times*, 23 October 1984.

15. Data Collection and Evaluation Unit, Public Health Program, Los Angeles County Department of Health Services, "Prenatal Care Attendance Patterns Study, June 1982." Contained in LA County Health Alliance et al., *Factual Memorandum and Argument in Support of Petition for Rulemaking*, 1984.

16. C. Hobel, Harbor-UCLA Medical Center, Department of Pediatrics and Obstetrics, in LA County Health Alliance et al., p. 14.

17. J. Merl, "Uninsured Must Pay $700 Deposit at County Hospitals," *Los Angeles Times*, 2 June 1982.

18. Ibid.

19. Capital needs estimate based on correspondence to the author from county officials in March 1984.

20. W. T. Price et al., "The 1982 Medi-Cal Reforms in Los Angeles County: The Implementation and Initial Impact of AB 799, AB 3480, and SB 2010" (Unpublished paper, May 1983), p. 6.

21. Ibid., p. 13.

22. See sources cited in n. 8 and N. Lurie et al., "Termination of Medi-Cal Benefits: A Follow-up Study One Year Later," *New England Journal of Medicine* 314 (8 May 1986): 1266–68.

23. M. R. Cousineau and E. R. Brown, "The Implementation of the Ability of Pay Plan for Uninsured Low Income Ambulatory Care Patients in Los Angeles County Department of Health Services" (Unpublished paper, August 1985).

24. Unpublished data supplied by Los Angeles County Department of Health Services.

25. Y. Honkawa, "The Nature of the Rate-Setting Mechanism and its Impact on the Public-General Hospital," in Commission on Public-General Hospitals, ed., *Readings on Public-General Hospitals* (Chicago: Hospital Research and Educational Trust, 1978), p. 446.

26. A. C. Roark, "USC May Have For-Profit Teaching," *Los Angeles Times*, 20 November 1984.
27. California Welfare and Institutions Code, SI7000.
28. "Board Policies Underlying the Planning for and Operation of the Department of Health Services for the Period 1984–1989" (Los Angeles County Department of Health Services), Exhibit 2-1.
29. Ibid.
30. Price et al., "Medi-Cal Reforms," p. 26.
31. Urban Institute, COTH Database.

# ✣ 5 ✣

# Hillsborough County Hospital Authority

## Joel Weissman and Martha Solish

The residents of Hillsborough County in Florida are served by two local public hospitals—Tampa General Hospital and Hillsborough County Hospital. Both are operated by the Hillsborough County Hospital Authority (HCHA), a public benefit corporation. In the recent era of local fiscal conservatism and increased competition from other area hospitals, HCHA has faced serious problems. This chapter examines the efforts of HCHA to remain viable in a changing and uncertain environment. The analysis focuses on the effect of two key events—the establishment of HCHA in 1980 and the agency's acute fiscal problems in 1983. HCHA's responses to these events afford a unique opportunity to examine how changes in governance structure and financing arrangements can affect a public hospital's performance.

## Background

**Organizational History**

Tampa General Hospital (TGH) was originally constructed in 1927 on Davis Island in Tampa Bay, a high-income, residential neighborhood. Its initial 250-bed capacity was expanded several times as the community grew; capacity reached 611 beds in 1982. A new construction program launched in that year raised the bed complement to 1,000 when the hospital's newest building opened in 1986.

TGH provides a wide range of services, including several that are not available at other hospitals in the county.[1] It has one of eight specialized neonatal care units in the state and one of four burn centers. It has a pediatric emergency room, a kidney transplant unit, and a 60-bed comprehensive physical rehabilitation center. In addition to these specialized services, TGH also provides a relatively large volume of more routine care to many of the county's indigent — for example, TGH's 49-bed obstetric unit provides care for practically all births to poor women in the area.

Hillsborough County Hospital (HCH) was constructed during the mid-1930s in a blue-collar community in the northeast section of Tampa. It comprises long, single-story wards and has 157 licensed beds, of which 80 are allocated to medicine and 77 to psychiatry. Its medical unit provides lower-cost placements for difficult dispositions and other longer-term cases transferred from TGH. HCH's psychiatric beds are reserved primarily for patients eligible for funding under the state's Baker Act, which assists non-Medicaid-eligible residents without private means to pay for psychiatric care. The facility accounts for over one-third of the Baker Act beds in Hillsborough County and is the only hospital in the area with such beds that provides a full range of medical services.[2] HCH also operates an extended-hours walk-in clinic that provides primary care to many local residents.

Together, the two HCHA hospitals constitute the largest inpatient facility in the county, accounting for over one-fifth of available beds. In 1984, the latest year for which data are available, HCHA facilities accounted for 23 percent of the 767,536 acute care days in Hillsborough County hospitals and about 10 percent of the nearly 500,000 outpatient clinic visits in the county.[3]

Prior to 1980, the county government operated both of Hillsborough County's public hospitals directly. The overall authority for general county government is the board of county commissioners, currently a seven-member group, four members of which are elected by district and three members of which are elected at large. Before 1984 the board consisted of only five members, all of whom served on the Hillsborough County Health and Welfare Board (HWB). The HWB was assigned oversight responsibility for social welfare functions, including the public hospitals. The HWB, in turn, appointed as executive director of the Hillsborough County Division of Hospitals the person who was the chief administrator for both TGH and HCH.

This governance arrangement was widely criticized as inefficient and ineffective. The county commissioners who served on the HWB were not selected for their interest or expertise in the health care field and had to devote their attention to numerous other civic issues as well. Responding to their concerns, the board of county commissioners created a five-member hospital council. The council consisted of private citizens with expertise in the health care field who would advise the county commissioners on health care matters and provide a link between the commissioners and the hospitals' executive director.

This revised governance structure served to complicate rather than alleviate the problems, because it created multiple levels of authority. The executive director had to go through two approval procedures for all major decisions. Budget and contract decisions had to be approved by the hospital council and then by the commissioners acting as the HWB. In addition, operation of the hospitals as a unit of county government subjected some staff decisions to patronage pressures and placed other employment decisions under civil service constraints.

In an effort to improve hospital operations, the county commissioners engaged an outside consultant. The consultant's 1979 report recommended creating an independent authority to run the hospitals. This proposal met no significant resistance, and state charter established HCHA in 1980. The quasi-public nature of HCHA carried with it certain obligations. The Authority is subject to the Sunshine Law, which mandates open meetings, and the board may only enter into contracts and endeavors that "serve the public good." The original legislation required HCHA to abide by county civil service requirements. This provision was later amended by state legislation to exempt the Authority from what were viewed as restrictive personnel policies, requiring instead that an employee advisory committee be established to represent staff previously protected by civil service.

The governing board of HCHA consists of nine members, including two county commissioners, the five private citizens who served on the hospital council, and two additional members. The HCHA board is responsible for setting long-range policy, approving all basic budget and program decisions, and reviewing all major contracts. The Authority has no taxing power, and so remains dependent on the county for subsidies to cover care to the indigent. The board of county commissioners retained full authority to determine the basis and amount of any subsidies from the county to HCHA. However, beyond deciding on an appropriate subsidy, the county commissioners exercise no operational oversight with regard to HCHA hospitals.

One of the new board's first priorities was planning and financing a major expansion and rehabilitation program. In 1982 HCHA issued $160 million in revenue bonds to finance a six-stage capital program that included a new physical rehabilitation center, an addition to TGH to increase its bed capacity to 1,000, and a 100-suite professional office building for medical staff. Repayment of principal on the bonds was to begin in September 1985.

## Table 5.1

### HCHA Operating Expenses and Revenues, Fiscal Years 1980–85 (dollars in thousands)

| | 1980 | 1981 | 1982 | 1983 | 1984 | 1985 |
|---|---|---|---|---|---|---|
| Operating expenses | $62,273 | $76,713 | $93,278 | $114,055 | $101,489 | $118,961 |
| Revenues | | | | | | |
| Patient service (net)[a] | 60,343 | 75,055 | 86,837 | 92,949 | 95,778 | 115,803 |
| Other operating | 2,483 | 2,502 | 2,849 | 3,282 | 3,560 | 3,715 |
| County subsidy[b] | 3,020 | 4,761 | 4,814 | 5,355 | 6,011 | 5,980 |
| Other nonoperating[c] | 888 | 1,789 | 1,317 | 511 | 183 | 1,597 |
| Total revenues | $66,734 | $84,107 | $95,817 | $102,097 | $105,532 | $127,095 |
| Surplus (deficit) | 4,461 | 7,394 | 2,539 | (11,958) | 4,043 | 8,134 |

Source: HCHA annual financial reports for FYs 1980–85.
[a]Includes payments by the county for indigent services (see Table 5.5).
[b]Excludes payments by the county for indigent services (see Table 5.5).
[c]Includes interest income in all years and loss on security portfolio restructuring of $582,000 in 1984.

In its 1983 fiscal year, HCHA incurred an operating deficit of about $12 million, or about 10 percent of its operating expenses (see Table 5.1). Since the Authority had previously generated operating surpluses and had been projected to continue to do so in order to repay its bonds, the deficit was a major source of concern. Although proposals were made to abolish HCHA and return the hospitals to county control, a solution was ultimately developed that improved the agency's finances. Operating expenses were reduced through several measures, including a layoff of 367 employees in August 1983. In addition, based on the recommendations of a task force under the auspices of the Greater Tampa Chamber of Commerce, a local sales tax of .25 percent was enacted, with the funds earmarked for HCHA. Following these measures, the Authority returned to a record of annual operating surpluses and now appears able to meet scheduled debt payments.

Medical staff arrangements for the hospital have been relatively stable since 1969, when a formal affiliation was developed with the newly opened University of South Florida (USF) Medical School. Before this affiliation, TGH sponsored residency programs that were supervised by community physicians with admitting privileges. Originally, local physicians supported the formation of a "hometown" medical school in Tampa. They looked forward to the prestige that a medical school affiliation would bring to TGH, and many anticipated receiving faculty appointments.[4]

However, the USF affiliation has been a source of tension in the local medical community since its inception. Instead of drawing faculty predominantly from among physicians already practicing in the area, the USF recruited its faculty largely from outside Tampa. The local physicians practicing at TGH resented this and sought to retain their authority within the hospital.

The result of these tensions is a relatively small teaching program and a dual medical administrative structure. As noted in Chapter 2, the ratio of residents to beds at HCHA is lower than that at the other public hospitals considered in this volume. In addition, the ratio of residents to adjusted patient days at TGH (5.7 per 10,000) is below that at other urban public teaching hospitals in the South (7.6) and nationwide (9.1).[5] The relatively limited medical school involvement in the hospital is also evident in the medical committee structure. The hospital functions almost as if it had two separate medical staffs—USF faculty and community physicians—each with its own committees. Most department chiefs are private practitioners; only obstetrics, pediatrics, general surgery, and otolaryngology are headed by full-time faculty. In some specialties (for example, ophthalmology), residents are supervised only by private physicians; in others, USF faculty teach but do not head the sections; and in some departments (radiology, pathology), exclusive agreements have been signed with private physician groups, effectively excluding USF faculty from practicing at TGH.

In July 1985, a new affiliation agreement was approved in an attempt to mediate the needs of USF faculty, private physicians, and HCHA administrators. The agreement established explicit communication mechanisms for the first time, including a joint affiliation committee, provisions for joint policy meetings, and physician representation on planning and review committees. It calls for TGH's medical director to receive a joint appointment as assistant dean at USF, providing a strong administrative link. It is important to note that the agreement does not grant USF the right of first refusal on all physician contracts, a right it had sought. Also, the medical staff bylaws were not amended to reflect the changes in the affiliation agreement. Nevertheless, this agreement represents a major step in improving medical staff relations.

### Regulatory Environment

The state of Florida has not sought to regulate closely its health care industry. Implementation of federal planning requirements and certificate of need procedures to regulate capital investments did not constrain the growth of hospital beds. HCHA had no conflict with local or state planning authorities over its planned renovation and expansion, despite the already high bed-to-population ratio in the area. The state also has not sought to regulate hospital payment rates, and HCHA, like other hospitals, has been able to shift costs to help fund indigent care.

However, the state has been concerned with controlling its expenditures under the Medicaid program, and three aspects of Florida Medicaid policy have been important to HCHA finances — eligibility rules, reimbursement limits, and revenue pools for uncompensated care. With respect to eligibility, Florida does not cover people in the medically needy category, restricting benefits to those receiving cash assistance, either Supplemental Security Income or Aid to Families with Dependent Children (AFDC). Moreover, the state-determined AFDC income eligibility limits are extremely low. For example, the federal poverty guideline in 1983 for a family of four was $10,200 while the Florida AFDC cutoff was $3,276. Consequently, relatively few of the poor qualify for Medicaid; in Hillsborough County, where approximately 90,000 persons were below the federal poverty level in 1981, there were only 6,918 active AFDC cases and 33,395 Medicaid recipients.[6]

Florida's Medicaid reimbursement policies limit hospital payments for both inpatients and outpatients. The program provides full payment only for the first 13 days of inpatient care; the 14th through the 45th days are provided at 65 percent of the full rate, and no payment is made after 45 days. Outpatient visits are paid at reasonable cost, but the state imposed a $100 annual limit per recipient in 1982, raising that limit to $500 in 1984.

Because the state's Medicaid program covers relatively few of the poor, there is a large poor, uninsured population that places a significant uncompensated care burden on hospitals in the state. To address this problem, the state adopted a new program in 1984 that created a public medical assistance trust fund. The fund's revenues are derived from a tax on hospital revenues, and these revenues are redistributed to hospitals in proportion to their volume of service to Medicaid patients. When the fund became fully operational in 1987, it was expected to provide an estimated net gain of $7 million to HCHA.[7]

## Trends in Performance

Events during the first half of the 1980s had a significant effect on HCHA's performance. The following sections trace the agency's standing in terms of efficiency, access, and quality.

## Table 5.2

## Comparative Measures of Efficiency, 1982

| | TGH | HCH | All Urban Teaching Hospitals in the South | All Urban Public Hospitals in the U.S. |
|---|---|---|---|---|
| Total staff per 10,000 adjusted patient days | 101.4 | 57.1 | 115.8 | 132.2 |
| Registered nurses per 10,000 adjusted patient days | 26.1 | 9.7 | 22.7 | 26.4 |
| Practical nurses per 10,000 adjusted patient days | 13.0 | 4.3 | 8.1 | 7.1 |
| Average salary per full-time-equivalent employee (in thousands of dollars) | $18.6 | $17.5 | $16.5 | $16.4 |
| Average salary per full-time-equivalent nurse (in thousands of dollars) | $14.1 | $15.4 | $20.1 | $19.6 |
| Payroll expense as a percentage of total expense | 48.9% | 53.2% | 51.7% | 51.0% |

Source: Special tabulation from the 1982 joint AHA–Urban Institute survey.

## Efficiency

By comparative standards HCHA appears to be an efficient system. Based on the regression model presented in Chapter 7 of this volume, the predicted cost per adjusted admission at HCHA was 66 percent above the actual cost. This suggests that after controlling for case mix, teaching intensity, and other factors, hospital management practices hold the actual unit costs below expected levels. Additional data indicating good comparative performance are HCHA's lower-than-average ratio of employees to work load and share of total expenses devoted to payroll (see Table 5.2).

However, during the 1980–84 period, HCHA declined in its relative efficiency (see Table 5.3). Total operating expenses per adjusted patient day increased 98 percent at HCHA during this four-year period; this is well in excess of the 78 percent and 68 percent increases at community hospitals in Florida and in the United States, respectively. It should be noted that the trend was concentrated in the first three years and that in 1984 HCHA's expenses rose more slowly than the reference group's, suggesting improvements in relative efficiency in 1984.

The decline in relative efficiency is related to large staff increases during the 1980–83 period. In a span of three years the number of full-

Table 5.3

Trends in Efficiency at HCHA Hospitals, 1980–84

| | 1980 | 1981 | 1982 | 1983 | 1984 | Percent Change 1980–84 |
|---|---|---|---|---|---|---|
| **Operating Expenses per Adjusted Patient Day** | | | | | | |
| HCHA (amount) | $ 269 | $ 329 | $ 391 | $ 500 | $ 533 | |
| HCHA (percent change) | — | 22.3 | 18.8 | 27.9 | 6.6 | 98.1 |
| Florida state and local acute care hospitals (percent change) | — | 14.7 | 18.8 | 12.3 | 14.3 | 74.9 |
| All Florida community hospitals (percent change) | — | 16.6 | 16.5 | 13.4 | 15.9 | 78.5 |
| U.S. state and local acute care hospitals (percent change) | — | 14.6 | 13.9 | 11.5 | 11.6 | 62.4 |
| All U.S. community hospitals (percent change) | — | 16.0 | 15.1 | 12.8 | 11.3 | 67.7 |
| **Full-Time-Equivalent Employees** | | | | | | |
| HCHA | | | | | | |
| Tampa General | 2,115 | 2,233 | 2,437 | 2,748 | 2,340 | 10.6 |
| Hillsborough County | 289 | 275 | 284 | 303 | 246 | -14.7 |
| Total HCHA | 2,404 | 2,508 | 2,721 | 3,051 | 2,586 | 7.6 |
| **Full-Time-Equivalent Employees per Adjusted Average Daily Census** | | | | | | |
| HCHA | 3.8 | 3.9 | 4.2 | 4.9 | 5.0 | 30.5 |
| Florida hospitals | 3.9 | 4.0 | 4.2 | 4.1 | 4.3 | 10.3 |
| U.S. hospitals | 3.4 | 3.5 | 3.8 | 3.6 | 4.4 | 29.4 |

Sources: Unpublished data from HCHA; *Statistical Guide*, 1980–1984 editions (Chicago: American Hospital Association, 1981–1985).

time-equivalent employees at HCHA increased by 647, or nearly 27 percent, while work load as measured by adjusted patient days actually fell slightly. HCHA's growth in employment-to-work-load ratio far exceeded the national average during this three-year period, and even continued in 1984 because work load fell more rapidly than employment.

## Access

Historically, Tampa General Hospital and Hillsborough County Hospital have provided most of the hospital care to the poor in their areas. In 1983, HCHA accounted for approximately 70 percent of bad debt and 56 percent of charity care among hospitals in the county.[8] In the same year, HCHA provided 61 percent of all Medicaid patient days provided in the county, although it accounted for only 26 percent of all county patient days.[9]

However, HCHA provides relatively less indigent care than do other urban public hospitals. Between 1980 and 1984, HCHA's charity care and bad debt averaged 16.5 percent of total charges, compared to 25.2 percent among all urban public teaching hospitals in the South.[10]

During the 1980–84 period, HCHA reversed its policies and performance with respect to access. From 1980 to 1982 both total services and care to the poor generally increased; then, in 1983 and 1984, HCHA reduced its total service volume, largely as a result of cutbacks in services to the poor.

The turnaround in service volume is evident for all major types of service (see Table 5.4). For inpatient services, discharges and patient days increased moderately from 1980 to 1982, then fell 16 percent and 18 percent, respectively, in the next two years. Outpatient services went from a 3 percent increase to a 40 percent drop in the two periods.

Most of the reduction in service was for indigent patients. The volume of bad debt and charity care had grown from 15.3 percent to 19.6 percent of gross revenues between 1980 and 1983; in the next year it fell to 17.0 percent as the absolute dollar value of deductions for bad debt and charity care was reduced for the first time in HCHA's history.

The reductions in access resulted from policy decisions made in August 1983, when the agency's financial problems became widely known, to deny nonemergent care to uninsured indigent patients. The Authority's enabling legislation provided that "no person in need of immediate or emergency treatment shall be denied admission to Tampa General because of an inability to pay."[11] However, the definition of emergency treatment had never been clarified. A new board policy discontinued unfunded elective surgery and limited the definition of emergency to situations in which there is a risk of death within 24 hours without treatment. As justification, the Authority chairman stated, "Those unfunded patients clearly belong to someone else — they are not our patients."[12]

The new policy was implemented by requiring prior approval from the county for all elective treatment to uninsured indigents. Alternatively, an uninsured patient could make a deposit that covered at least 80 percent of the estimated cost of the procedure.[13] A $50 deposit was required for nonemergent care provided in the emergency room.

## Quality

The limited available evidence indicates that HCHA provides relatively high quality care and that there was no significant change in

## Table 5.4
## HCHA Service Volume, Fiscal Years 1980–84

| | 1980 | 1981 | 1982 | 1983 | 1984 | Percent Change 1980–82 | Percent Change 1982–84 |
|---|---|---|---|---|---|---|---|
| Patient discharges | | | | | | | |
| Tampa General Hospital | 21,916 | 21,873 | 22,331 | 22,284 | 19,115 | 1.9 | (14.4) |
| Hillsborough County Hospital | 2,275 | 2,366 | 2,213 | 1,798 | 1,417 | (2.7) | (36.0) |
| Total | 24,191 | 24,239 | 24,544 | 24,082 | 20,532 | 1.4 | (16.3) |
| Patient days | | | | | | | |
| Tampa General Hospital | 174,034 | 172,088 | 177,136 | 172,503 | 146,888 | 4.0 | (17.1) |
| Hillsborough County Hospital | 29,183 | 32,945 | 34,298 | 31,755 | 26,976 | 17.5 | (21.3) |
| Total | 203,217 | 205,033 | 211,434 | 204,258 | 173,864 | 4.0 | (17.8) |
| Outpatient services | | | | | | | |
| TGH outpatient visits | 39,588 | 41,964 | 43,429 | 28,469 | 23,345 | 9.7 | (46.2) |
| TGH emergency room visits | 58,050 | 57,750 | 57,088 | 54,347 | 38,021 | 1.7 | (33.4) |
| Hillsborough County Hospital | 30,162 | 30,758 | 31,200 | 28,946 | 17,681 | 3.4 | (43.3) |
| Total | 127,800 | 130,472 | 131,717 | 111,762 | 79,047 | 3.1 | (40.0) |

Source: HCHA annual report for FY 1984. Fiscal year is October 1 to September 30.

quality during the 1980–84 period. The January 1984 survey by the Joint Commission found no deficiencies in areas of medical services and awarded accreditation contingent only on the elimination of two deficiencies relating to the documentation (as opposed to delivery) of care. The deficiencies related to prompt completion of medical records and to delineation of clinical privileges in the emergency room. Both were subsequently remedied.

Interviews with members of the Tampa medical community not affiliated with HCHA also provided evidence of a high quality of care. These observers invariably cited Tampa General's specialized services and inferred that provision of tertiary services allowed for adequate continuity of care. An HCHA official commented that paying patients "come here only when they're really sick, but they stay," instead of transferring to a hospital with more amenities and better perceived quality of nursing care. The construction of new hospital facilities has contributed to a widely held community perception of high quality.

The only notable criticisms of quality were general impressions raised in a few interviews. One observer believed that "civil service is not conducive to delivery of good patient care" and therefore that the public system was inferior to others. Another criticism was that too few USF staff had been recruited to ensure adequate resident supervision, and that the staff "haven't had the support or inspiration to realize their potential."

## Governance and Financing

The history of HCHA illustrates how the transfer of a public function to a semiautonomous organization carries with it burdens as well as advantages. Shortly after its creation, HCHA had some notable accomplishments. However, the governance change also generated a lack of communication and eventual conflicts between the board of county commissioners and HCHA officials. These conflicts contributed to poor financial management and the fiscal crisis of 1983.

The crisis, in turn, precipitated another round of governance changes, including a more active HCHA board, a new chief executive officer, and the emergence of a watchdog task force at the chamber of commerce. The crisis also led to eventual increases in county support, including a new sales tax devoted to indigent care. In addition, the state increased its Medicaid payments and established a new program to aid hospitals serving the poor. Because of the new revenues and management efforts to curb expenditure growth, the HCHA's financial outlook improved. These later changes are related to the reductions in access and the improved efficiency that followed.

## Initial Benefits

Historically Tampa's public hospitals were in an unusually favorable financial situation. Because of TGH's location on affluent Davis Island and because of the support of community physicians, privately insured patients represented over half of TGH's admissions in the mid-1970s. Charges for these patients provided revenues sufficient to pay for a large portion of the indigent care the hospital provided. As a result, the necessary county subsidy was small, usually less than 10 percent of gross revenues. Moreover, the county subsidy generally permitted the public hospitals to have a modest operating surplus.[14]

This pattern of financing was gradually undermined during the 1970s. Between 1971 and 1978, admissions of privately insured patients to TGH declined over 37 percent.[15] The loss of appeal to private patients resulted from greater competition from newer private facilities being constructed in the area and the failure of the county to invest in new plant and equipment. The public facilities deteriorated, contributing to the decrease in the number of private patients.

The HCHA was established to provide more independent governance of the county hospitals. The advantages of the new agency were that one decision-making body would replace the fragmentation of the hospital council and the Health and Welfare Board; the decision makers would be people with a better understanding of the hospital industry and greater independence from local politics; and the Authority would have independent access to capital funds through the power to issue revenue bonds.

The creation of HCHA, with its independent borrowing authority, was seen as a way to reverse the declining situation. For several years the county had been unwilling to borrow to finance hospital construction because the commissioners did not want to raise the taxes needed to meet bond payments. With the creation of the Authority, the hospital leaders had independent access to capital funds, and they quickly planned a major expansion and renovation project. One of the HCHA board's first actions was to obtain a certificate of need for expansion and renovation. The HCHA board approved a bond issue in 1982 to finance the project. The Authority was able to act quickly on a hospital endeavor that had been perceived as needed for a long time.

The feasibility study for the bond issue projected that HCHA operating surpluses would grow from $6.7 million in 1983 to $24 million in 1988. The optimistic projections were based on increases in the number and share of privately insured patients, greater overall utilization due to rapid population growth in neighboring areas, and 9 percent annual growth in per diem rates.[16] In essence, expanded cost shifting and a growing number of private patients were expected to finance HCHA operations and capital programs.

The legislation creating HCHA also granted the agency a two-year exemption from civil service requirements. The expectation was that this would permit more efficient personnel practices. While there is no objective evidence that the hospital system became more efficient during HCHA's early years (see Table 5.3), observers reported that the new system improved morale. On these grounds the exemption was renewed.

The combination of improved employee morale and the launching of a major construction program enhanced the public hospitals' image in the community. There was an improvement in perceived quality of care that probably helped the hospitals attract more private patients in the long run.

### Conflicts and Fiscal Crisis

HCHA's initial record of accomplishment was significantly marred in 1983 when the agency incurred a large operating deficit and had to borrow to cover its expenses. While several factors led to the fiscal crisis, one important cause was a lack of policy coordination between HCHA officials and the board of county commissioners. HCHA engaged in a large expansion program at the same time the county was seeking to curb its expenditures for indigent health care; the result was conflict between the organizations over county funding levels.

As documented in Tables 5.1 and 5.3, HCHA management expanded budget and personnel significantly in its early years. From 1980 to 1982, operating expenses increased 50 percent and the number of employees grew by 317, or 13 percent. Service volume did not increase proportionately, suggesting that these new resources represented some combination of quality enhancements and reduced efficiency.

HCHA continued these resource expansions in 1983. Its operating expenses jumped over 22 percent as staff were increased by another 330 and additional salary increments were granted. At the same time, the county accelerated its efforts to curb spending for indigent hospital care. The principal mechanism for accomplishing this was to place low income limits on those eligible for county assistance and to impose rigorous requirements for documenting eligibility. Consequently, a

Table 5.5

County Support for HCHA, Fiscal Years 1980–85
(dollars in thousands)

| | 1980 | 1981 | 1982 | 1983 | 1984 | 1985 |
|---|---|---|---|---|---|---|
| County payments for<br>indigent patient services | NA | $5,212 | $5,868 | $5,679 | $6,800 | $9,300 |
| Subsidy for HCH | 1,588 | 3,153 | 2,862 | NA | 3,694 | 3,642 |
| Medical education<br>subsidy | 1,432 | 1,608 | 1,952 | NA | 2,317 | 2,338 |
| Proceeds of sales tax | — | — | — | — | — | 15,000 (est) |
| Total support | NA | 9,973 | 10,682 | 11,034 | 12,811 | 30,280 |

Sources: Office of the Auditor General, "Report on Audit of the Hillsborough County Hospital Authority" (State of Florida, 12 December 1983); HCHA, budget for FY 1985; HCHA, audited financial statements for FYs 1980–84.

NA: Not available.

growing source of conflict between HCHA and the county was the large and increasing number of patients rejected for county assistance after services had been provided. There was little coordination between hospital staff and county eligibility screening personnel. In fact, eligibility counselors were removed from TGH in July 1982, allegedly due to lack of space. This made eligibility certification during a patient's hospital stay nearly impossible.

As a result of these county policies, the county's payments to HCHA in 1983 fell far short of what the Authority had anticipated, and lagged the growth of previous years. County payments to HCHA for services to indigent patients actually fell 3 percent in 1983, compared to a nearly 13 percent increase in 1982 (see Table 5.5). The other forms of county subsidy partly offset this loss, but total county support increased only 3 percent in 1983 compared to over 7 percent the previous year.

County officials did not publicly deny responsibility for indigent care, and some admitted that the county had failed to live up to its commitment.[17] However, they also tried to shift the blame by raising issues of incompetence and inadequate planning by HCHA administrators, and suggested that indigent health care could be provided more efficiently by contracting with providers other than TGH and HCH.[18]

**Responses to the Crisis**

It is not clear when the HCHA board became aware of the extent of its fiscal problems and how promptly it responded. Communication between hospital managers and the board was not clear or complete. Financial reports were not issued regularly in the six months preceding the crisis, and budget status reports did not adequately inform the board of hospital financial operations. However, the inadequate reporting procedures cannot be blamed on management alone; the board did not seek the information that would have enabled it to oversee the agency's finances more competently. Moreover, once it became aware of the crisis, the board did not respond as quickly as it might have. In December 1983, Florida's auditor general issued a report charging that the Authority "knew of the Hospital's poor financial condition and failed to plan an adequate response."[19]

The first adjustments to the financial crisis were the restrictions on nonemergent indigent care described earlier and the layoff of 367 employees in August 1983. While the personnel cuts achieved some expenditure reductions, they also significantly reduced service volume and sacrificed revenues. From 1983 to 1984 there was a 29 percent drop in outpatient department and emergency room visits and a 15 percent drop in discharges (see Table 5.4). Apparently patients did not seek care, not wishing to be turned away.

Public pressure for additional action came in November 1983 when Standard and Poor's, a bond-rating agency, put HCHA bonds on a credit watch on the ground that HCHA's fiscal problems threatened its ability to pay debt service. In response, the board of county commissioners asked the local chamber of commerce to create a task force to consider the future of HCHA. In addition, the HCHA board replaced the executive director of TGH with an experienced administrator with impressive credentials, from a prestigious teaching hospital in Houston.

In the following weeks, HCHA's public image improved dramatically. The new director projected a sense of competent leadership.[20] He was primarily the beneficiary of felicitous timing, because the measures taken before his arrival were finally yielding some improvement in fiscal performance. But the new director effectively publicized the positive results, creating a new community confidence. The better performance alone probably would not have been sufficient to change the public image.

The creation of the task force also proved to be of long-run significance. The members were respected business community leaders with no direct involvement in either HCHA operations or county government. Thus they had both a new perspective and great public credibility. They also benefited from their ability to meet privately, a privilege not available to either the HCHA board or the county commissioners under Florida's Sunshine Law. This law prohibits any two members of a public board from meeting to discuss public business unless the press is notified and invited.

After examining the HCHA finances, the task force recommended in April 1984 two measures that provided substantial additional revenue. First, they recommended, and used their political contacts to help pass, a county sales tax increase of .25 percent that was earmarked for indigent hospital care. Second, they helped convince the county to increase its income standards for indigent care. This provided additional county funds to HCHA. The effectiveness of these measures was evident in HCHA's 1985 budget (see Table 5.5). The sales tax provided an increase in revenue of $15 million, and payments for indigent services jumped more than one-third, to $9.3 million. In all, county support more than doubled, from $12.8 million in 1984 to $30.3 million in 1985.

Although the task force completed its report in early 1984, it has continued to meet and serve as both advocate for and watchdog over HCHA. The success of the task force has been attributed to its exemption from the Sunshine Law and to its members' contacts in state and county government. It serves as a surrogate board in many ways, performing functions, such as setting strategic policy, that the actual HCHA board is constrained in performing by the Sunshine Law.

The success of the task force has led the HCHA board to consider converting HCHA to nonprofit status to avoid the requirements of the Sunshine Law. However, there are important drawbacks to this step. First, a nonpublic authority would not be protected by sovereign immunity and might be subject to significantly increased malpractice liability claims. Second, the authority could lose part or all of its county indigent care subsidy. Finally, the authority might lose any community support it derives from its role as provider of last resort to the poor.

In 1984, additional measures were taken to improve HCHA operations. A special management unit was established, and it developed a productivity monitoring system.[21] Employee education and morale seminars were begun in an effort to reduce overtime and improve productivity. Middle-level managers were transferred from hourly pay to salary to give them greater status and incentives. In the area of financial management, the previous 7- to 10-day average billing lag was reduced to 4 days in 1984, and accounts receivable were reduced significantly in that year.

These improvements resulted in a $12.6 million reduction in operating expenses between 1983 and 1984 and slowed the growth in expenses per adjusted patient day to 6.6 percent from 28 percent (see Tables 5.1 and 5.3). The layoffs and further staff attrition led to a 15 percent decline in full-time-equivalent employment in 1984. However, staffing per adjusted average daily census showed no improvement, since service volume declined at the same time.

In sum, the short-run responses to fiscal crisis were to reduce expenditures, primarily through staff reductions, and to secure additional county revenue. With the aid of the chamber of commerce task force, the HCHA obtained higher income eligibility levels for county-paid patients and secured passage of a county sales tax increase that earmarked approximately $15 million in annual revenue for HCHA. In addition, the passage of state legislation providing revenues for indigent care improved the long-run revenue picture.

The substantially increased county funds since 1984 and the later increases in state funds for indigent care represent an altered financial course for HCHA. Rather than relying more heavily on revenues from privately insured patients, the Authority has become more dependent on public subsidies. Its long-run ability to become competitive, and to repay its debt successfully, remains untested. In the future HCHA will still have to supplement its enlarged public sudsidies with substantial growth in private, third-party revenues.

It also is not clear whether the recent increases in HCHA's county and state revenues have reversed any of the efficiency improvements or access restrictions generated by the 1983 fiscal crisis. There are some indications that conditions are improving. Compared to previous years the new rehabilitation center is much more open to admitting indigent patients, and the HCH clinic is seeing more Medicaid patients.

## *Teaching Relationships*

### Current Situation

Medical staffing at TGH is divided between community physicians in private practice and faculty of the USF Medical School who combine teaching salaries with private practice income. The community physicians play a much stronger role in hospital affairs than do the medical school faculty, and the community physicians are primarily concerned with tertiary services while the medical school faculty's dominant interest is primary care. This pattern is unusual among urban public hospitals.

The strong position of community practitioners is due to their critical role in generating hospital revenues and to the financial and other weaknesses of USF. HCHA's long-run plans require TGH to be a tertiary care center with a large proportion of privately insured patients. To attract these patients the hospital needs community-based private practitioners.

However, private physicians have been leaving TGH in large numbers as a result of dissatisfaction with the administration and the attraction of new opportunities in private hospitals.[22] For example, in 1983 and 1984, two of the cardiac surgeons who had provided numerous lucrative cardiac surgery admissions moved to other hospitals.

HCHA has developed several initiatives to attract and retain private physicians. First, older facilities were renovated with the hopes of attracting some physicians to TGH. For example, the new trauma center is jointly staffed by USF and private physicians. Second, a new medical office building was constructed to provide office space for private physicians, and HCHA management planned to include enticements such as subsidized rent, equity shares, and guaranteed practice income for physicians with new practices. Finally, efforts were made to increase efficiency in the admitting and medical records departments in order to respond to a history of complaints from private physicians wishing to admit and follow their patients.

In contrast, HCHA views USF faculty as tied to a financially weak institution and as a source of competition for private patients on both an individual and an institutional basis. USF is the newest and smallest of Florida's three medical schools and widely perceived as underfunded relative to the other schools. USF's teaching program at TGH is the only such program that requires a county subsidy because it is not fully funded by the state. The chamber of commerce task force report of 1984 recommended that the state make a larger contribution in order to reduce necessary county funding.

As is true in many medical schools, the USF faculty seek to supplement their salaries with private practice income. However, the strong presence of private practitioners at TGH creates bitter battles. The private practitioners accuse faculty of stealing patients, while faculty members complain that HCHA administrators do not understand their need to make money and resent being expected to provide almost all the uncompensated care. Also, the relatively low faculty salaries associated with state underfunding have caused high faculty turnover. Faculty members who leave often set up private practices in the local community, generating additional competition for insured patients.

The USF Medical School as an organization is also viewed as a potential source of competition. This feeling of competition is tied to USF's expansion plans, which include a 140-bed cancer treatment and chronic disease hospital and a number of other facilities on the USF campus. The medical school leadership claims that the cancer hospital will not divert patients from TGH. However, there is a great deal of concern among TGH's community physicians that general acute care services will be provided at the new USF hospital and that it will be used to serve insured patients, leaving indigent care to be provided at TGH.

In addition to funding problems and perceived threats of competition, the specialty orientation of USF faculty generates conflict with TGH's community-based practitioners. In most teaching hospitals, community physicians are likely to be primary care practitioners who refer patients to university faculty for specialty care. At TGH, the reverse is true. Private practitioners dominate the complex specialty departments, while USF faculty are predominantly in primary care fields. In fiscal year 1984, as Table 5.6 shows, private practitioners accounted for over 80 percent of all TGH admissions in cardiology, nephrology, and cardio-thoracic surgery; USF faculty provided 98 percent of all pediatric and 96 percent of all obstetrics/gynecology admissions.

The long-range plan of HCHA is to expand tertiary care in pursuit of prestige and profitable, privately insured patients. In contrast, the priority orientation of USF faculty is primary care. USF faculty have proposed, for example, the establishment of a family practice residency at TGH. Thus, TGH private practitioners and USF faculty are pulling the hospital in opposite directions.

**Implications of Current Policies**

Large teaching programs and strong medical school affiliations have been hypothesized to lead to higher unit costs, greater provision of care to the poor, and higher quality of care. TGH is an unusual example of a public hospital with a relatively small teaching program and weak medical school links; therefore, it provides an opportunity to explore the hypothesized relationships from a distinct vantage.

With respect to efficiency, HCHA does have adjusted unit costs substantially below its peer groups (see Chapter 7). This supports the hypothesis that greater teaching commitment leads to increased unit costs. However, the fluctuations in relative efficiency at HCHA in the 1980–84 period seem unrelated to shifts in teaching policy. While the general trend has been for university faculty to account for more admissions, this trend has not decreased relative efficiency. Instead, HCHA's improved efficiency in the post-1983 years seems tied to changes in financing that reduced available resources.

The weak academic links are consistent with the sharp reductions in access following the 1983 fiscal crisis. The reduction in outpatient and other services to the indigent probably affected primary care ser-

## Table 5.6

### Admissions to Tampa General Hospital, Fiscal Year 1984

| Specialty | Number of Admissions | Percentage by University Faculty | Percentage by Private Practitioners |
|---|---|---|---|
| General surgery | 1,653 | 53.7% | 46.3% |
| Orthopedics | 1,253 | 80.1 | 19.9 |
| Cardiology | 1,415 | 13.4 | 86.6 |
| Nephrology | 805 | 18.6 | 81.4 |
| Pediatrics | 5,789 | 98.0 | 2.0 |
| Cardio-thoracic | 1,388 | 8.4 | 91.6 |
| OB/GYN | 1,945 | 95.7 | 4.3 |
| All others | 4,872 | 58.8 | 41.2 |
| Total | 19,120 | 66.7% | 33.3% |

Source: Unpublished data from HCHA.

vices disproportionately. Thus, despite the USF faculty's strong interest in primary care and its responsibilities for indigent care, a major response to reduced resources was to cut such services. This reflects the weak role of USF in setting hospital policy.

Although teaching affiliations are often linked to high standards of quality for specialty services, this is not clearly the case at HCHA. USF faculty do not supervise all the teaching services associated with high-technology medicine; in the services for which USF provides supervision, the small faculty size often prevents adequate supervision. While TGH apparently gains some status because of its medical school affiliations, the more significant lesson from the HCHA case is that high quality tertiary care at a public hospital can be obtained through reliance on community physicians as well as on medical school faculty.

## Market Strategy

### Current Strategy

Although HCHA did not have a formal strategic plan during the case study period, a coherent plan guided the creation of the Authority and many subsequent actions of its board. HCHA intended to capitalize on its unusual base of private practitioners by expanding the volume of services to privately insured patients. Revenues from these services would be sufficient to help fund indigent care and keep necessary county subsidies to a minimal level. To accomplish these goals, the

Authority would initiate a major capital program, promote tertiary care programs, and pursue other policies to attract community physicians with private practices.

This strategy seemed viable and desirable to county officials when HCHA was created. However, developments in the early 1980s posed threats to its future viability. The rapid expansion of competing institutions made HCHA's strategy more difficult to follow. Between 1981 and 1984, construction of 800 additional beds was authorized in Hillsborough County.[23] Sixty-nine applications for major construction projects were received by the state in 1982, more than in the previous eight years combined.[24] Among the new projects were several that provided a direct competitive threat to HCHA. St. Joseph's Hospital opened two open-heart-surgery units and two cardiac catheterization units and staffed them by drawing away two of TGH's three cardiac teams. (The cardiac program had been TGH's major profit center). University Community Hospital sought approval for open-heart surgery and cardiac catheterization units as well.

As a result of growing competition from expanding hospitals and a larger supply of private practice physicians, HCHA has not been successful in enhancing its market position. HCHA furnished 26 percent of all patient days in the county in 1984, down from 28 percent in 1980. Market shares of specialty services such as open-heart surgery and cardiac catheterization are leveling off or declining. The services for which HCHA has a relatively high share of the county total are rehabilitation (73 percent), obstetrics (37 percent), and psychiatry (48 percent).[25] For several of these services, notably obstetrics, most of the patients are poor residents rather than privately insured, middle-class patients.

Heightened competition limited HCHA's ability to obtain added revenues by cost shifting. TGH has historically been a relatively expensive facility, and its capital program has added to costs. Thus there has proved to be little room for higher charges as other hospitals have begun price competition efforts.

Other factors also have raised problems for the initial market strategy. TGH's location is becoming a market weakness as most population growth takes place on the north side of Tampa. The HCHA board's inability to meet confidentially, due to the Sunshine Law, has limited its ability to plan effectively. Finally, the continuing indigent care responsibilities perpetuate the last-resort image of HCHA's facilities.

To cope with these increasingly difficult circumstances, some new efforts have been made. The opening of newly constructed facilities has enhanced TGH's image in the community. To attract privately insured patients, HCHA is emphasizing the quality improvements it has achieved through renovation and special programs like CARE (an acronym for courtesy, attention, respect, and efficiency), established to train the nursing staff to meet higher standards when dealing with privately insured patients and the physicians who admit them. To promote price competitiveness, charges at TGH were held constant from October 1983 to October 1985. HCHA's hope is that more competitive prices will encourage newly formed preferred provider organizations in Florida to develop ties with TGH.

### Implications of Current Strategy

HCHA's implicit market strategy can be related to its performance during the case study period. The large expansion of staff and increased operating expenditures during 1980–83 may have reflected the desire to enhance operations in order to attract more privately insured patients. While it is difficult to distinguish the resulting inefficiencies from the gains in quality, it is likely that the expenditure growth of that period reflected some reductions in efficiency. In this sense the combination of a new governance structure and a competitive market strategy can be linked to lower efficiency.

Similarly, these two factors facilitated the decision to reduce access in response to the financing changes and the 1983 fiscal crisis. The reduction in services to the indigent was consistent with a market strategy that gave first priority to bringing in more privately insured patients.

It is likely that the capital program and expanded staff funded in HCHA's early years improved quality of care. However, competition for private patients led HCHA to assign a low priority to its teaching affiliations with USF. To the extent that such academic affiliations enhance quality (and the extent is questionable in USF's case), this may be interpreted as a possible negative factor.

## Summary

The creation of HCHA in 1980 marked the beginning of a turbulent period for Tampa's public hospitals. During the next five years HCHA completed a major capital project, experienced a financial crisis, and weakened its resolve to be the provider of last resort for the poor.

HCHA was created to facilitate financing of capital improvements, to expand managerial freedom, to reduce political influence, and to improve the hospitals' public image. The quick passage of the bond issue was a good beginning for the fledgling organization. The change in governance, therefore, was closely associated with new capital improvements, which created a perception of improved quality of care.

But the governance change alone did not affect efficiency or access. Managers continued to complain of an inefficient, civil-service mentality, and political appointees remained on the HCHA board and in the hospital administration. The HCHA board was initially unable to curb the rapid rise in expenditures, and its policies continued to permit a growing volume of uncompensated care to the indigent.

Only when changes in financing arrangements were coupled with the new governance structure were more dramatic changes in performance evident. Clearly the governance change signaled an effort to create political distance between the Authority and the board of county commissioners. It also created a gap in accountability. HCHA was no longer beholden to the county board except for a small proportion of its revenues. Furthermore, repaying the bond debt and establishing a favorable position in the credit market had taken precedence among the concerns of the HCHA board. In turn, the county commissioners felt that the financial health of the public hospitals was no longer their responsibility and limited the flow of county funds to HCHA. The commissioners believed that HCHA could and would subsidize internally the costs of providing care to indigent patients. The HCHA board believed that it required operating surpluses to repay debt and upgrade its services and that it was responsible for serving only those indigents for whom it was adequately paid.

These conflicts in policy between HCHA and the board of commissioners (together with Medicaid reductions and other external factors) led to a fiscal crisis in 1983, when HCHA experienced a $12 million operating deficit and had its bonds placed on a credit watch by a rating agency. The new governance structure influenced HCHA's responses to this crisis. The HCHA board improved efficiency by cutting personnel and restricted access by denying care to indigent patients. In this sense, the combination of a reduced local subsidy and more independent governance led to both greater efficiency and reduced access.

HCHA was also created to follow a competitive market strategy. This led to its initial emphasis on improving its hospitals' public image. In relatively successful media campaigns, it emphasized new physical plant. The image of the hospital system as a wasteful and unresponsive operation gradually improved to that of an efficient and modern system offering highly specialized care.

Competitive strategies generally are not conducive to access for the poor. Uncompensated care for indigent patients must be financed by increases in the price of services to insured patients; this causes the hospital to become less price-competitive. The response of HCHA to its fiscal crisis supports this connection. Nonetheless, the administration at HCHA believes this shortcoming is outweighed by the benefits of competition. The recent capital improvements and anticipated improvements in efficiency and image are expected to benefit everyone, including the indigent.

The effect of HCHA's weak teaching affiliation with USF on hospital performance is indirect and often mixed. HCHA needs USF faculty and house staff to bolster its tertiary care image, but the lack of comprehensive supervision of house staff in certain departments brings into question whether the USF affiliation enhances quality for all specialties. With respect to access, USF faculty are responsible for care of virtually all indigent inpatients. However, the weak affiliation and the financial needs of the faculty reduce their influence at HCHA; the faculty's interests have not been sufficient to offset pressures for reduced access caused by financing and governance changes.

## *Notes*

1. Information on specialized services in the state of Florida is from "Financial Feasibility Study" (Tampa: Price Waterhouse, 24 September 1982).
2. Information on Baker Act services is from "Report to HCHA" (Joint Review Committee on Hillsborough County Hospital, 1 January 1985).
3. "1984 Annual Hospital Utilization Report" and "Primary Health Care Component" (Health Councils of West Central Florida, 1984).
4. Hillsborough County Hospital has 26 active medical staff members, all of whom are USF faculty. HCH's only teaching program is in adolescent psychiatry. Therefore, the teaching issues discussed in this chapter relate primarily to TGH.
5. Figures are unpublished tabulations from "Survey of Medical Care for the Poor and Hospitals' Financial Status, 1982" (Joint survey of the American Hospital Association [AHA] and the Urban Institute).
6. Personal communication from Florida Department of Health and Rehabilitative Services, 20 January 1986.
7. Memorandum (Florida Hospital Association, 15 October 1984).
8. "Financial Data Report" (Florida Hospital Cost Containment Board, 1983).
9. "1984 Annual Report" and "Primary Care Component."
10. Figures are unpublished tabulations from the 1982 joint AHA–Urban Institute survey.
11. Laws of Florida, Chapter 80-510.
12. Marilyn Kalfus, "Indigent Care May be Cut by Hospital," *Tampa Tribune*, 14 September 1983.

13. Office of the Auditor General, "Report on Audit of the Hillsborough County Hospital Authority" (State of Florida, 12 December 1983).
14. Health and Institutional Consultants, "Executive Summary: Management and Operations Audit, Division of Hospitals, Hillsborough County" (Kurt Salman Associates, February 1979).
15. Marilyn Kalfus, "TGH Feeling 'First Breeze' of Progress," *Tampa Tribune*, 7 May 1984.
16. "Financial Feasibility Study" (Price Waterhouse).
17. Alan Sverdlik, "Hospital, County Officials Squabble over Care for Poor," *Tampa Tribune*, 19 August 1983.
18. Alan Sverdlik, "Request for Bailout Defeated," *Tampa Tribune*, 14 August 1983.
19. Office of the Auditor General, "Report on Audit of the HCHA."
20. Kalfus, " 'First Breeze' of Progress."
21. "Annual Report, Fiscal Year 1984" (Hillsborough County Hospital Authority), p. 3.
22. "Report of the Tampa General Hospital Task Force" (Greater Tampa Chamber of Commerce, 3 April 1984), p. 40.
23. Ibid.
24. Alan Sverdlik, "Tampa General Fights for Share of Patients," *Tampa Tribune*, 20 March 1983.
25. "District Health Plan" (Health Councils of West Central Florida, 1984).

# ⚜ 6 ⚜

# The Regional Medical Center at Memphis

## Mary G. Henderson

The Regional Medical Center in Memphis, Tennessee (the Med) is an example of an urban public hospital in transition. Previously known as the City of Memphis Hospital, in 1981 it changed from being operated as a unit of county government to governance by a not-for-profit corporation. Additional changes include an increased concentration in some areas of tertiary care and the construction of new facilities, the most prominent being a regional trauma care center.

At the same time the Med has striven to alter its service mix and upgrade its image, the hospital has retained its strong commitment to care for the poor and uninsured (including many patients from outside Shelby County). The hospital faces a major challenge in balancing a potentially more profitable service mix against the primary care needs of its indigent patients. The hospital also has reevaluated its strong teaching affiliation with the University of Tennessee College of Medicine. This relationship increases the hospital's prestige and quality of care; it also increases costs, reduces public control over services, and limits relationships with community physicians. Cutting across many of these issues is the Med's position as the predominant source of care for indigent blacks in a racially polarized city. Given this fact, it is not clear whether the Med can become a community hospital with broad appeal. This chapter focuses on the problems a public hospital faces as it tries to become more economically viable while maintaining its mission of care to the poor.

# Background

### Organizational History

Shelby County is the unit of local government responsible for providing public health services to the approximately 777,000 people living in Memphis and the adjacent suburbs that make up the county. In fiscal year 1986, Shelby County allocated nearly $50 million, or 20 percent of its operating budget, for medical care. Of that money, 72 percent, $35.8 million, went to the Med. A smaller portion, $3.5 million, was spent on acute care services for children through a contract with LeBonheur, a pediatric hospital. The remaining $10 million was divided almost equally among health centers providing ambulatory care and two county-operated nursing homes.[1]

Established in 1829, Memphis's public hospital was the first hospital in Tennessee. As the City of Memphis Hospital, it was managed as a unit of county government by a volunteer board appointed by the mayor of Shelby County. In the late 1970s, it sustained persistent and increasing operating losses. County officials threatened to decrease their financial support and questioned whether a new construction project (already funded) should take place, given the lack of a plan to fund the resulting increased operating expenses. A widely shared view in local political and business circles was that the volunteer board, known as the Memphis–Shelby County Authority, was not governing the hospital adequately.

The failure of the volunteer board to govern the hospital effectively was often attributed to the intrusion of elected officials in the affairs of the hospital. The appointed board members were not able to act independently of the Shelby County government in many significant ways. Basic decisions about purchasing, personnel policies, contracts, and labor union matters came before meetings of the county commission.

The formation of the Shelby County Health Care Corporation (SCHCC) was perceived as a last-ditch effort to save the hospital. With the support of business leaders and the county board of commissioners, this separate not-for-profit corporation was formed on June 15, 1981. It is empowered to own and operate health facilities, including the Med. However, the Med still relies heavily on its county appropriation to cover its significant annual operating deficits.

The Med is affiliated with the University of Tennessee College of Medicine (UT), which offers medical training in 19 specialties throughout the state. In 1985, the Med accounted for 133 of UT's 384 full-time clinical faculty and 136 of the 491 residencies UT supervised. The largest residency training programs were in obstetrics/gynecology, general surgery, and other subspecialties of internal medicine.[2]

Although UT utilizes the Med as its primary teaching facility, much of the care at the hospital is routine obstetrical, medical, and surgical. UT is the largest single provider of maternity care in the county, with 45 percent of all live births in the county occurring there in 1983. The hospital's ratio of births to admissions (39.9 births per 100 admissions) is more than twice as high as those of other urban teaching hospitals located in the South.[3] The occupancy rate for the obstetrics/gynecology service is among the highest of all services.[4]

Many complicated therapeutic and diagnostic procedures are not performed at the Med. In 1980 specialized cardiac procedures were transferred to the William F. Bowld Hospital, a 162-bed tertiary care hospital. The Bowld Hospital is housed in a building UT now owns but had leased from the SCHCC until 1985. Over three-quarters of the Med's surgical procedures are performed on an outpatient basis, a much higher proportion than at other area hospitals.[5]

Although much of the care the Med provides is routine, the hospital recently began to offer specialized services in the areas of neonatal, high-risk maternal, trauma, and burn care. Med administrators market these "centers of excellence" to appeal to privately insured patients. Drawing on its excellent reputation as the high-volume provider of newborn specialty care in the county, the Med has expanded its obstetrics service to include midwifery and alternative birthing arrangements.

The Med's ability to market its centers of excellence depends on a $61 million expansion and renovation program financed by general obligation bonds issued by Shelby County. The major component of this project is the Elvis Presley Trauma Center, begun in 1979 and completed in 1983. This facility, the only major trauma center in the region, is staffed by teams from the UT faculty.

The Med operates 450 of its 620 licensed beds. It annually provides approximately 19,000 admissions and 132,000 patient days, which account for about 10 percent of all admissions and patient days in Shelby County. The hospital provides approximately half of all uncompensated (bad debt and charity) hospital care in Shelby County. About 50 percent of the Med's charges are for uncompensated care.[6]

The Med provides more outpatient care than the other hospitals in the county. In 1985, about 36 percent of all hospital outpatient department visits in Shelby County were provided in the 27 general and subspecialty clinics at the Gailor Outpatient Clinic, which is staffed by UT faculty, interns, and residents. Other hospitals offer outpatient care primarily to patients referred to specialty clinics by physicians. Although the Med's share of county outpatient care remains large, the number of visits declined 27 percent (from 118,455 to 86,887) between 1980 and 1984. Factors accounting for this decline include the transfer of pediatric clinics to LeBonheur, the closing of specialty clinics, and the opening of an outpatient clinic at Bowld. Recently, however, the number of outpatient visits has begun to increase.[7]

Emergency room visits at the Med declined 16 percent (from 62,852 to 52,951) over the 1980–84 period but increased as a proportion of all such visits in the county, from 22 percent to 28 percent, in the same period.[8] As is the case with clinic visits, utilization of the Med's emergency room has increased recently; between 1984 and 1985 visits grew 9 percent. There is substantial inappropriate use of the emergency room because many indigents cannot afford private doctors for nonemergency ailments, because the community perceives the emergency room as the place to go for all types of care, and because the diagnostic capabilities of the county's community health centers are severely limited.

### Regulatory Climate

Because it is the primary hospital for the indigent of Shelby County, the Med's financial condition is strongly linked to the nature of the state's Medicaid program. Unfortunately, Tennessee has one of the nation's most restrictive Medicaid programs. While nationally about 53 percent of individuals with incomes below the poverty level are eligible for Medicaid, in Tennessee only 28 percent are eligible. Moreover, the average payment per recipient is approximately 15 percent below the national average.[9]

The low Medicaid payments result largely from limitations on inpatient hospital benefits. Before 1983, Medicaid covered 20 days of inpatient care per recipient per year; new regulations in 1983 reduced this to 14 days. In 1982, Tennessee's medically needy program was also functionally eliminated for non–nursing home services. Although pregnant women and children with special disabilities are eligible to qualify through the spend-down provision, few do qualify because the state's asset and income eligibility levels are among the lowest in the nation.

Although eligibility and benefits are restricted, Tennessee Medicaid payments to hospitals are more generous. The average payment per inpatient day in Tennessee was $285 in 1984, about 9 percent below the national average. However, a new payment system became effective in 1984 and is more favorable to hospitals, including the Med.

In 1984, the Med received an average per diem payment of $708, higher than its costs.[10] Reimbursements for physician services and for outpatient care are also higher than those in many other states' Medicaid programs.

Fortunately for the Med, the special problems confronting large public hospitals are receiving increased attention at the state level. In April 1984, Tennessee increased its Medicaid coverage for certain groups, including pediatric patients, from 14 to 20 inpatient days per year, and there is pressure to reinstate 20 days of inpatient coverage for all recipients. In addition, the new hospital payment system initiated in 1984 provided extra funds to hospitals serving an exceptionally large proportion of Medicaid patients. As noted above, these reimbursement changes have had favorable financial consequences for the Med.

Another feature of Tennessee's regulatory climate is a new disposition against planning. In 1985, a select committee on health care cost containment in Tennessee endorsed competition as the best long-range strategy for controlling costs. The committee specifically called for phasing out the certificate of need program. During the transition phase, the committee recommended that the CON authority be used to pursue opportunities for bed reductions. This recommendation is guiding the current policy of the health planning agency. After determining that the bed-to-population ratio in Shelby County was more than double the ratio required, the agency called for bed reductions as part of any construction project.

## Trends in Performance

The Med's performance varied among the three criteria during the 1980–84 period. The hospital appears to have become less efficient, to have maintained a relatively high level of access to care by the poor, and to have improved the quality of its services.

### Efficiency

At the start of the 1980s, the Med's cost per adjusted day ($363) was well above the comparable figures for community hospitals both in the state of Tennessee and in the nation (see Table 6.1). Similarly, the ratio of employees to work load was substantially higher at the Med than the statewide or national average. Moreover, the statistical model presented in Chapter 7 indicates that the cost per admission was 23 percent higher than expected, given the hospital's case mix and other relevant factors. While not conclusive, these data strongly suggest that

## Table 6.1

## Trends in Efficiency at the Med, 1980–84

|  | 1980 | 1981 | 1982 | 1983 | 1984 |
|---|---|---|---|---|---|
| **Operating Expenses per Adjusted Patient Day** | | | | | |
| The Med (amount) | $363 | $326 | $285 | $453 | $556 |
| The Med (percent change) | — | (10.2) | (12.6) | 58.9 | 22.7 |
| Tennessee state and local acute hospitals (amount) | $183 | $216 | $241 | $268 | $319 |
| Tennessee state and local acute hospitals (percent change) | — | 18.2 | 11.8 | 11.2 | 19.1 |
| All Tennessee community hospitals (amount) | $204 | $241 | $275 | $299 | $344 |
| All Tennessee community hospitals (percent change) | — | 18.1 | 14.3 | 8.9 | 15.1 |
| U.S. state and local acute hospitals (amount) | $239 | $274 | $312 | $348 | $388 |
| U.S. state and local acute hospitals (percent change) | — | 14.6 | 13.9 | 11.5 | 11.6 |
| All U.S. community hospitals (amount) | $245 | $294 | $327 | $369 | $411 |
| All U.S. community hospitals (percent change) | — | 20.0 | 11.2 | 12.8 | 11.3 |
| **Full-Time-Equivalent Employees** | | | | | |
| The Med | 2,453 | 2,116 | 1,994 | 1,986 | 2,250 |
| **Full-Time-Equivalent Employees per Adjusted Average Daily Census** | | | | | |
| The Med | 5.0 | 4.5 | 4.4 | 4.2 | 5.1 |
| Tennessee hospitals | 3.2 | 3.2 | 3.3 | 3.3 | 3.9 |
| U.S. hospitals | 3.4 | 3.5 | 3.8 | 3.6 | 4.4 |

Sources: Unpublished data from the Regional Medical Center at Memphis and data from the *Statistical Guide*, 1980–1984 editions (Chicago: American Hospital Association, 1981–1985).

the Med began the case study period as a relatively inefficient institution.

However, the available data also indicate that the Med's relative efficiency improved somewhat. From 1980 to 1984, average cost per adjusted day increased 53 percent at the Med, compared to 69 percent for community hospitals in Tennessee and 68 percent for hospitals nationwide. The gain in relative efficiency was due to an absolute reduction in unit costs in 1981. In subsequent years, the rate of

## Table 6.2
## Utilization of the Med, 1980–84

|  | *1980* | *1981* | *1982* | *1983* | *1984* | *Percent Change 1980–84* |
|---|---|---|---|---|---|---|
| Admissions | 20,554 | 19,387 | 17,658 | 17,765 | 16,956 | (17.5) |
| Patient days | 134,696 | 128,610 | 125,054 | 112,788 | 104,948 | (22.1) |
| Occupancy rate | 77.8% | 76.6% | 81.8% | 73.7% | 81.4% | 4.6 |
| Average length of stay (days) | 6.6 | 6.6 | 7.1 | 6.3 | 6.2 | (6.1) |
| Outpatient visits | 118,455 | 103,309 | 97,507 | 94,506 | 86,887 | (26.6) |
| Emergency room visits | 62,921 | 77,530 | 70,622 | 67,485 | 66,194 | 5.2 |
| Total ambulatory care visits | 181,376 | 180,839 | 168,129 | 161,991 | 153,081 | (15.6) |

Source: Unpublished data from the Regional Medical Center.

increase in the Med's unit costs was higher than the comparable state-wide and national figures. This relatively poor performance in the later years can largely be attributed to declines in utilization that were not matched by budget reductions (see Table 6.2). During the 1980–84 period, patient days fell over 22 percent and ambulatory care visits declined nearly 16 percent.

## Access

Consistent with its mission, the Med provides a substantial amount of care to the uninsured. Between 1980 and 1984, the Med's bad debt and charity care deductions accounted for 45 percent of the total of such deductions in Shelby County ($185.6 million out of $431.6 million), although the hospital accounted for only 8 percent of total acute care patient days.[11] The Med's bad debt and charity care remained high throughout the study period, approximately half of gross patient revenues. Payer mix information also discloses a high proportion of care provided to Medicaid and self-pay patients (see Table 6.3). Data on payer mix of ambulatory care patients indicate that over half are "self-pay/no-pay" patients.[12]

Despite the overall decline in utilization, the Med has maintained a high level of access for the indigent. The volume of care to Medicaid and uninsured patients is estimated to be nearly stable in the face of an aggregate drop in patient days. That is, nearly all the decline in utilization was among the Medicare and commercially insured patients. Between 1980 and 1984, the share of patient days represented by

## Table 6.3

### Patient Days by Payer at the Med, Fiscal Years 1980–84

| | *Percentage of Days* | | | | |
| | *1980* | *1981* | *1982* | *1983* | *1984* |
|---|---|---|---|---|---|
| Medicare | 22% | 19% | 17% | 16% | 16% |
| Medicaid | 23 | 29 | 30 | 28 | 26 |
| Commercial insurance | 16 | 12 | 12 | 12 | 12 |
| Self-pay and other | 39 | 40 | 41 | 44 | 46 |
| Total | 100% | 100% | 100% | 100% | 100% |

Source: Unpublished data from the Regional Medical Center.

Medicare patients fell from 22 percent to 15 percent and the share represented by self-pay patients rose from 39 percent to 46 percent.[13]

## Quality

The Med's predecessor, the City of Memphis Hospital, suffered from the image of an institution providing low quality service. The hospital had a deteriorating physical plant, and many observers believed that the quality of care was substandard. Staff were viewed as inattentive and impolite to patients. Despite the excellent reputation of its emergency room, the hospital generally was viewed as "not clean, not private, not desirable."

Upon gaining control of the hospital, the SCHCC began many initiatives to upgrade the Med that could potentially affect quality of care. Nevertheless, based on Joint Commission surveys in 1984 and 1985, several problem areas remained. In the 1984 report, the Med's three-year accreditation was made contingent upon compliance with a set of recommendations in 14 major areas, most of which involved deficiencies in quality assurance. The report found evaluation, monitoring, and documentation of patient care to be inadequate. In addition, it identified major quality assurance problems concerning the delineation and performance of medical staff roles. Another major concern was nursing services, where licensed practical nurses and vocational nurses often substituted for registered nurses. Finally, buildings and grounds safety problems were uncovered, particularly in two antiquated buildings used in patient care (although accreditation was not made contingent upon the correction of these deficiencies).

Because of the large number of recommendations cited in its 1984 report, the Joint Commission conducted a focused survey one year later. It found that the medical staff and quality assurance areas now satisfied requirements but that problems remained in the areas of peer review and documentation. The Joint Commission warned that the Med's accreditation status would be jeopardized unless the hospital evidenced substantial compliance in these areas through written progress reports. By 1985, the hospital had met the required contingencies and the Med received a valid three-year accreditation from the Joint Commission.

## *Governance*

### Current Structure

The SCHCC is a not-for-profit corporation established by Shelby County. It has an agreement with the county to provide acute inpatient care at the Med. The president of the hospital is an ex officio member of the 12-member SCHCC board and reports directly to the board. A significant change in the new governance structure is that the president of the hospital is responsible for the day-to-day operations of the hospital.

Although decisions regarding daily operation can now be made independently by the president, the county still maintains a significant measure of control. The county subsidy accounts for almost one-third of the Med's annual operating costs, and the county funds almost all capital investments. The mayor of Shelby County appoints the members of the SCHCC board, subject to the approval of the county board of commissioners (an 11-member elected body). Thus this board, which selects the president, is heavily influenced by the county. Two board committees, the executive committee and the finance committee, are primarily responsible for overall policy and planning, personnel decisions, and budget approval.

### Initial Effects of the Governance Change

The Med's new governing structure became effective on 1 July 1981. At that time, the SCHCC awarded a management contract to Methodist Hospital Management, Inc. (MHM). This firm, a subsidiary of another Memphis hospital corporation, had no experience in running a public hospital with a large indigent care responsibility. Indeed, one reason it was selected was its promise to draw privately insured patients.

The management firm performed poorly. Between 1982 and

1983, commercially insured admissions actually decreased from over 14 percent to 12 percent of total admissions. Self-pay admissions rose from 36.6 percent of the total in 1982 to 40.2 percent in 1983.[14] To some extent, factors beyond MHM's control contributed to these changes in payer mix. These factors include the previously discussed tightening of Medicaid eligibility, a downturn in local economic conditions, and a rise in medically indigent transfers from other area hospitals. Hospital staff calculated that nearly 100 indigent patients per month were transferred to the Med from the emergency rooms of the privately owned Memphis hospitals.[15]

Management problems for which MHM was more directly responsible include inadequate record keeping, which led to overcharges that were discovered by Medicaid and Medicare audits, and a large increase in charges in 1983 that served to discourage the commercially insured patients. Additionally, the hospital's fiscal and administrative service expenses doubled in MHM's first year. Finally, although MHM claimed it could manage the hospital with a $22 million county subsidy, it required $26.7 million and an emergency appropriation from the county in 1983.

Despite these performance problems, MHM initiated a number of positive changes. The quality of financial and other management information improved at the hospital. The reorganized hospital received the support necessary from the county commissioners and the business community to continue the funding of the new construction.

In addition, when the new SCHCC did not reduce access to care by the indigent, the black community accepted and supported the reorganization. An important factor in this acceptance involved UT, widely regarded in the black community as a "lily-white" institution. The new governance structure was perceived as being able to gain more control over the Med-UT relationship, an ability the black community applauded.

**Recent Effects of the Governance Change**

The role of MHM was reduced to a consulting function in 1984. Since that time, in-house managers have gained in credibility. They have enhanced financial control systems, begun to address productivity concerns, and upgraded the nursing staff. In 1984, almost 300 full-time-equivalent personnel, mostly registered nurses, were hired to staff the new trauma center. Management has acted on recommendations from the Joint Commission review team to reduce the proportion of licensed practical nurses, and no licensed practical nurses have been recruited since 1984.

Based on Joint Commission results as well as on interviewee comments and numerous newspaper articles, it appears that quality of care at the Regional Center has improved since the reorganization and especially since 1983. The image of the hospital has also significantly improved, and this has raised staff morale. It is difficult, however, to separate the effects of new governance from the effects of the construction projects, since both changes transpired during the same time period. As mentioned above, though, the county's continued willingness to fund the expenses of the capital projects was largely due to the governance change.

Although quality improvements have been made and relationships with significant groups in the community have improved, major problems remain. Administrators are concerned about low employee productivity and lack of staff responsiveness to patients and managers. There are significant personnel problems, including high absenteeism, sick leave abuse, and functional illiteracy among the unskilled staff. In 1984, an action plan was implemented to improve employee productivity and morale. The plan included management effectiveness training, communications workshops, and a "pay for performance" system. The plan also provided for a productivity committee of union representatives and hospital administrators. Salary increases depended on reduced absenteeism. Since the plan was instituted, absenteeism has been reduced from 6 to 5 percent, but it is still well above the industry standard of 2.5 percent. The new management is perceived as driving a harder bargain with the union, but because the county is responsible for negotiating contracts with the local union, the direct role of the Med administration is attenuated. Additionally, because the union employees are mostly black, there are sensitive political and racial issues involved in improving productivity.

Although the current administration of the Med remains hopeful that the image of the hospital can continue to improve and that the Med can begin to draw more paying patients, the governance changes instituted since 1981 are not likely to be sufficient to cause such changes. The primary problem is the financially poor patient mix that underlies the poor financial condition of the hospital and continues to reinforce the hospital's image as the black, indigent care hospital. It is important that the new governance structure improve relationships with the county, because the hospital needs the county subsidy to cover a substantial portion of its operating expenses. This subsidy has remained relatively stable since 1982 at $26 million, and it will need to remain at least at that level for the next several years.

## Teaching Affiliation

Memphis's public hospital has been affiliated with the University of Tennessee College of Medicine since 1926. This long relationship has benefited both parties. The hospital has obtained a complement of residents and staff physicians to provide care; the medical school has obtained a place to train its doctors and to pursue its research interests.

As in most relationships between public hospitals and medical schools, however, there has been some conflict. The problems among the county, the hospital, and UT surfaced after 1977 when the county began to pay UT for managing the hospital and for medical staff services. UT's management proved unsatisfactory, and soon neither the hospital board nor the county commissioners saw UT as serving the interests of the hospital or the county. An ill-conceived plan to manage the hospital as a regional referral center for all population groups called UT's management expertise into question. Indigent black patients and the black community did not trust UT, felt that UT did not treat patients appropriately, and resented the use of black indigent patients as teaching material. Even after the county again assumed management control in 1981, relations between UT and the hospital remained tense when the SCHCC began managing the hospital.

### Current Situation

Over 130 graduate medical and dental interns and residents from UT provide services to patients at the Med. Faculty instruct and supervise the house staff and perform other medical and administrative duties on 16 separate medical services. Although in principle non-UT physicians can admit to the Med, in practice this happens only rarely because house staff will not see their patients. This situation has contributed to bad feeling in some parts of the black community where UT is perceived as a bastion of white-dominated medicine that prevents black community physicians from admitting to the Med.

Since 1982, the affiliation agreement between UT and the Med has been amended each year, underscoring the changing nature of the relationship. Over the years, the SCHCC has become a stronger force in negotiating this agreement. The Med's payments to UT have decreased from over $15 million in fiscal year 1981 to $12.7 million in 1986. This is at least partially due to the Med's insistence that UT become more accountable in documenting patient care activities.[17] Additionally, the new contract explicitly states that patients seen at clinics at the Med be referred to the Med for inpatient and further outpatient care regardless of payer. This provision attempts to prevent the referral of paying patients to the Bowld or other area hospitals.

The Med administration and the dean of UT undertake policy decisions jointly. One decision that illustrates the delicate balance of power between the hospital and the medical school concerned the appropriate role and orientation of the medical director at the Med. UT preferred that the director be a faculty member and report to the dean. Some members of the SCHCC board wanted the medical director to report to the board and be stationed at the Med in order to prevent the director from becoming a UT "insider." The final resolution in 1985 called for the director to be an employee of the Med, reporting to the president. However, he also was a UT faculty member whose salary was paid by both the Med and UT. The role of the medical director, therefore, is seen as one element of an overall strategy to balance the interests of the hospital and the medical school.

The UT teaching affiliation is seen as a critical component of the Med's strategy to upgrade its image and capitalize on its centers of excellence. The medical school was instrumental in convincing the county to finance the new construction at the hospital to make it a place that could attract paying patients and one in which the medical school's interns and residents could provide care to a more financially mixed patient population. The Med needs its affiliation with UT in order to provide a broad range of tertiary care specialties and to staff its centers of excellence. Thus, despite problems, the Med and UT have an interdependent relationship that benefits both.

**Continued Conflicts**

Although the relationship between UT and the hospital has improved under the SCHCC, some disagreements remain. These have crystallized in two areas: the UT physicians' practice of billing privately insured Med patients separately under a nonprofit professional corporation called the University Physicians Foundation (UPF) and the UT physicians' continued use of the Bowld Hospital to treat their privately insured patients.

In addition to what the Med pays UT under its contract to provide services to indigent patients at the Med, UT receives two other kinds of payment from the Med and its patients. The hospital pays the full price for services to Shelby County indigents treated at the Bowld (over $2 million in fiscal year 1986), and the UPF collects an additional (currently unknown) amount from the Med patients and third parties.[18] The Med administration is currently pressing for disclosure of the amount UT collects from private patients, with an eye toward renegotiating the indigent care contract.

The UPF is a nonprofit professional corporation that is responsible for generating approximately half of all the salary income of the over 200 UT clinical faculty in 34 medical school departments. The remainder of UT's salary expenses is paid primarily through state taxes. The UPF physicians, therefore, have a strong incentive to provide fee-for-service medicine to paying patients. This mission conflicts with that of the Med, which is to provide health care to the indigent. It is ironic that the development of the centers of excellence, a process strongly supported by the Med, has increased the need to generate salary income to pay for the research and for the higher-priced medical staff required for the centers.

One illustration of the UPF physicians' desire to generate income from private patients is the introduction in 1986 of a "private wing" that aims to keep private patients who enter through the trauma center from transferring to private hospitals as soon as their condition is stabilized. Although not yet an active source of controversy, the fact that the "best and friendliest" staff are used in this unit may further highlight the areas of the hospital that are not as well served — the medical and surgical units — which have the highest proportion of black indigent patients.

The UT currently owns and operates the Bowld Hospital, and UT faculty use it as a private practice facility. It emphasizes highly specialized services like kidney and liver transplants, nuclear cardiology, and arterioplasty. Some of these services were previously available at the Med, but they were transferred to the Bowld in 1980. The county traded the Bowld to UT for an older, less well-equipped hospital as a goodwill gesture in the late 1970s, when private practice at the Med was not considered a viable alternative.

The availability of the Bowld has led to a "creaming" phenomenon — privately insured patients are referred to the Bowld while indigent patients go to, or remain at, the Med. In 1985, the Med had less than 10 percent of its admissions paid for by Medicare, while at the Bowld one-half of the admissions were Medicare patients. In contrast, one-third of the Med's admissions were reimbursed by Medicaid, compared with less than 7 percent of the Bowld's admissions.[19] Further, because of the Bowld's service mix, it is seen as skimming high-margin patients in need of intensive and technologically based services.

As mentioned earlier, under the current affiliation agreement, patients who are seen in clinics at the Med are admitted to the Med regardless of payment source. However, the UPF physicians continue to make direct referrals to Bowld (as well as to other private Memphis hospitals) in the belief that privately insured patients would not wish to receive inpatient care at the Med. This practice, in addition to house staff's not seeing patients referred to the Med by local practitioners, exacerbates the problem of attracting and retaining private patients. Thus, while the UPF physicians are siphoning off the commercially insured to the Bowld and other hospitals, local physicians whose patients receive Medicaid or are privately insured are deterred from using the Med.

The Med and UT administrators are working to reach a modus vivendi on the role of the Bowld and other problem issues. They are seeking to develop ways to encourage UPF physicians to have private patients choose the Med. Med administrators are also reevaluating how much UT is paid to provide indigent care, and UT officials are considering proposals to move some specialized services back to the Med. Considering that the Med needs its affiliation to retain its new image of higher quality and to provide services in its centers of excellence, while UT values the Med as a place to train interns and residents, both parties are motivated to arrive at a satisfactory arrangement.

## Financing

Like many urban public hospitals, the Med finds its major financial problem is that too many of its patients have inadequate or no medical insurance. As the only public hospital in the region, it serves as the hospital of last resort for the residents of Shelby County and parts of the neighboring states of Arkansas and Mississippi. To the extent that the Med continues to fulfill its mission of caring for all, regardless of ability to pay, its finances will remain heavily dependent on a county subsidy. This dependence on a subsidy from local government has important implications for the hospital's limited capacity to improve its performance.

### County Subsidy and Appropriations

Since 1980, county subsidies have covered a substantial portion of the hospital's operating needs. As shown in Table 6.4, however, the county has stabilized its operating subsidy at about $26.7 million since fiscal year 1983. As a result, the subsidy has covered a declining proportion of the Med's operating expenses, which have steadily increased since 1981. This has resulted in difficulties in meeting working capital

## Table 6.4

## Revenues and Expenses of the Med, Fiscal Years 1980–84 (dollars in thousands)

|  | 1980 | 1981 | 1982 | 1983 | 1984 |
|---|---|---|---|---|---|
| Expenses |  |  |  |  |  |
| Nursing services | $21,387 | $16,988 | $19,960 | $21,048 | $25,496 |
| Other professional services | 22,378 | 22,852 | 22,673 | 23,659 | 25,608 |
| General services | 12,628 | 9,391 | 8,705 | 9,862 | 10,624 |
| Fiscal and adm. services | 6,706 | 5,485 | 10,858 | 11,577 | 11,870 |
| Depreciation and amortization | 2,187 | 2,066 | 2,029 | 2,390 | 4,915 |
| Interest | – | – | 124 | 900 | 1,172 |
| Total operating expenses | $65,286 | $56,782 | $64,349 | $69,436 | $79,685 |
| Contractual services for indigent patients | 449 | 2,037 | 2,162 | 2,356 | 2,362 |
| Total expenses | $65,735 | $58,819 | $66,511 | $71,792 | $82,047 |
| Revenues |  |  |  |  |  |
| Operating revenue | $38,608 | $31,592 | $41,035 | $37,625 | $53,701 |
| Net county appropriation | 23,656 | 19,740 | 20,028 | 26,680 | 26,700 |
| Total revenue | $62,264 | $51,332 | $61,063 | $64,305 | $80,401 |
| Excess of expenses over revenues | $3,471 | $7,487 | $5,448 | $7,487 | $1,646 |

Source: Regional Medical Center annual reports for FYs 1980–84.

needs (its ratio of current assets to current liabilities was under 1.0 in three of the past five years) and in deficits.

In addition to providing the operating subsidy, the county is responsible for almost all capital expenses, including the $60 million hospital expansion and renovation project begun in 1979. The capital improvement appropriations averaged $3 million annually between fiscal years 1981 and 1985. A further recurrent county expense, estimated at over $6 million annually, is for interest to retire debt for the Med construction in prior years. (Although the county assumed responsibility for debt service, the Med still claims interest expense and depreciation as reimbursable expenses.) Finally, the surplus of $5.6 million in 1985 was a result of Shelby County's forgiving a debt of $8.6 million. If this had not occurred, the Med would have reported a deficit of almost $3 million in that fiscal year.

### Operating Expenses

An analysis of the Med's operating expenses indicates that many of the increases observed since the advent of the SCHCC have been due to improvements in staffing and the hospital's physical plant. Depreciation expense more than doubled between 1983 and 1984, and nursing services expenses rose more than 21 percent in the same period (see Table 6.4). The former expense increase was due to the major building and renovation project, while the latter was due to the hiring of over 200 nurses, mostly registered nurses, to staff the trauma center. Although these expense increases appear to be justified on the basis of quality improvements, some others are not as easily explained.

Fiscal and administrative expenses almost doubled between 1981 and 1982 while the hospital was being managed under the MHM management contract. Some of the current Med administration who were interviewed questioned the reasonableness of this rise in expenses. These costs have stabilized, however, since the new management has assumed control.

Although the Med has been understaffed in terms of registered nurses, it is considered to be overstaffed with less-skilled employees. Among nonfederal Shelby County hospitals, the Med is the lowest in terms of personnel costs per full-time staff person ($19,593 in fiscal year 1985) but third highest in personnel costs per licensed bed ($76,238 in fiscal year 1985).[20] The only two hospitals with higher personnel costs per bed are specialty and research hospitals. As mentioned earlier, the Med's number of full-time employees per average adjusted daily census (5.1 in 1984) is also high relative to other southern teaching hospitals. One administrator has said, "There is as much concern about the Med being a place to provide employment as there is concern for the Med to provide patient care." Another has said, "We could cut the payroll costs tomorrow."[21] Absenteeism and a liberal sick-day policy have increased personnel costs by contributing to a high ratio of paid days to worked days.

The Med's cash flow problems have also contributed to higher expenses. Lack of available cash (as indicated by accounts payable that remain unpaid for longer than desirable time intervals) means that the Med is unable to take advantage of discounts for timely payments. In addition, vendors may not consider the Med as a preferred customer eligible for special prices.

## Indigent Care

Indigent care has had very significant financial implications for the Med. Patient days not reimbursed through commercial or governmental insurance increased from 39 percent of total days in 1980 to 46 percent in 1984. Although the proportion dropped to 40 percent in 1985, the first 10 months of 1986 witnessed a rise to 46 percent.[22]

The Med made a few token attempts to impose restrictions on charity care to cut its operating losses. The hospital attempted to limit dumping in 1982 by stating that it would not accept transfers if their acceptance would prevent emergency patients from being treated. In 1983, the Med tried to require clinic deposits and deposits for prescription drugs on the second visit. Also in 1983, the hospital stated that it would impose limits on treatment of out-of-county Tennessee residents. None of these restrictions was effectively enforced, however, and all had little or no effect on transfers, utilization, and the number of out-of-county indigents treated. Their implementation did serve to publicize the hospital's plight, and some documentation of the problem emerged as a result.

**Future Prospects**

The Med's future financial prospects depend mainly on its primary source of funds, the county. Although the level of the operating subsidy has remained constant at $26.7 million since 1983, the county continues to contribute heavily to the Med's capital costs. When the amount the county pays to retire the Med's construction debts is added to what it pays for capital and operating subsidy, total payments to or for the Med in fiscal year 1987 are estimated at $38 million. Thus the Med is no less dependent on the county than it was before the SCHCC assumed control of the hospital.

It is increasingly unlikely that the Med will be able to achieve a profitable payer mix. The proportion of admissions with commercial insurance is estimated at 14 percent for fiscal year 1986, no different than the actual proportion for 1982. Medicare and Medicaid admissions have actually declined slightly over the same interval (Medicare from 9.3 to 8.4 percent; Medicaid from 34.0 to 32.8 percent).[23] The Med will continue to require significant public support to continue to carry out its indigent care mission. The recent changes in the state Medicaid program, which have increased coverage and allowed a disproportionate share adjustment for high-volume Medicaid providers, are signs of greater public awareness of the problem and support for the hospital. The county has also recently appointed a task force on indigent care, which will consider reorganization of county health services. In addition, discussion is taking place in the press as to whether indigent care costs should be shared by not-for-profit hospitals.

Although the volume of indigent care is not decreasing, some positive financial signs began to appear as a result of the new construction. Commercial insurance revenue increased 57 percent between 1984 and 1985, growing from 22 percent to 26 percent of total revenues.[24] Commercial payments rose both because of the high intensity of care provided in the trauma center (the average bill is reported to be around $100,000) and because the patients are likely to have full insurance coverage for trauma care. Thus, the county-financed construction is yielding some positive financial results for the Med.

## Market Strategy

As is increasingly the case with many public hospital systems, the Med is attempting to fulfill its mission of caring for the poor while simultaneously seeking to attract privately insured patients. The SCHCC has tried to balance these two goals, with mixed success. As discussed in the last section, the Med is obtaining a larger share of its revenues from privately insured patients but uninsured patients still dominate its payer mix in terms of admissions and patient days. To many people in Memphis, the hospital is still identified as the City of Memphis John Gaston Hospital, opened in 1936 to provide indigent care to Negroes. This hinders its acceptance as a community hospital that caters to the insured of all races.

### Current Market Position

Fourteen nonfederal hospitals are located in Shelby County (see Table 6.5). In 1983, the Med had the fifth highest number of beds in the county. The Med, with 7 percent of the staffed beds, experienced 10 percent of inpatient admissions and provided 8 percent of total patient days. The Med has increased its market share since 1983. Its operational beds have increased by almost 3 percent while all other nonfederal hospitals decreased theirs by 5 percent. The Med's share of total admissions has risen to 12 percent and its share of total patient days has grown to 10 percent. (See Table 6.6.) As discussed earlier, however, this growth is not made up of patients with commercial insurance; the proportion of total admissions covered by commercial insurance rose less than 2 percent from 1983 to 1985.

Utilization has grown at the Med, while declining at other area hospitals. The Med's inpatient admissions have increased since 1982. From 1980 to 1982, admissions dropped 14 percent, from 20,554 to 17,658. From 1983 to 1985, admissions rose more than 15 percent, climbing from 18,354 to 21,166. As Table 6.6 shows, this trend was not observed in Shelby County hospitals as a group; total nonfederal admissions declined over 5 percent in these hospitals over the same period. The same pattern is observed for patient days, for which the

## Table 6.5

## Short-Term General and Special Hospital Utilization in Shelby County, 1983

| Hospitals by Auspice | Admissions | Staffed Beds | Patient Days | Average Census | Occupancy Rate | Average Length of Stay | Births |
|---|---|---|---|---|---|---|---|
| **Municipal** | | | | | | | |
| The Med | 18,354 | 399 | 126,798 | 359 | 84.1 | 6.9 | 7,342 |
| **State** | | | | | | | |
| UT/Bowld | 4,019 | 126 | 31,755 | 87 | 66.4 | 7.9 | 0 |
| **Nonprofit** | | | | | | | |
| Baptist Memorial | 59,169 | 1,949 | 592,250 | 1,450 | 74.1 | 10.0 | 5,101 |
| B'nai Brith | 189 | 10 | 1,825 | 5 | NA | 9.6 | 0 |
| Harris Memorial | 7,092 | 174 | 53,290 | 146 | 83.9 | 7.5 | 0 |
| LeBonheur Children's Medical Center | 11,452 | 152 | 48,910 | 134 | 88.2 | 4.3 | 0 |
| Methodist South | 7,746 | 174 | 54,020 | 148 | 85.1 | 7.0 | 0 |
| Methodist Central | 31,698 | 892 | 277,765 | 761 | 80.2 | 8.8 | 2,200 |
| St. Francis | 24,495 | 663 | 197,465 | 541 | NA | 8.1 | 1,090 |
| St. Joseph's | 9,610 | 440 | 103,295 | 283 | 64.3 | 10.7 | 743 |
| St. Jude's | 1,722 | 48 | 10,585 | 29 | 60.4 | 6.1 | 0 |
| **Proprietary** | | | | | | | |
| Eastwood | 4,108 | 140 | 31,755 | 87 | 62.1 | 7.7 | 0 |
| Humana Specialty | NA | 50 | NA | NA | NA | NA | NA |
| Mid-South | 2,667 | 190 | 40,880 | 112 | 58.9 | 15.3 | 0 |

Source: *1984 Guide to the Health Care Field* (Chicago: American Hospital Association, 1985).

Note: Totals do not include hospitals for which data were not available (NA). Data are not shown for psychiatric or long-term care hospitals.

## Table 6.6

## Trends in Operational Beds, Admissions, and
## Patient Days in Shelby County, 1983-85

|  | 1983 | 1984 | 1985 | Total Change | Percent Change |
|---|---|---|---|---|---|
| **Operational Beds** | | | | | |
| The Med | 426 | 437 | 437 | 11 | 2.6% |
| All nonfederal hospitals in Shelby County | 5,576 | 5,486 | 5,311 | (265) | (4.8) |
| **Admissions** | | | | | |
| The Med | 18,354 | 19,382 | 21,166 | 2,812 | 15.3% |
| All nonfederal hospitals in Shelby County | 182,355 | 181,614 | 172,703 | (9,652) | (5.2) |
| **Patient Days** | | | | | |
| The Med | 126,798 | 132,039 | 139,142 | 12,344 | 9.7% |
| All nonfederal hospitals in Shelby County | 1,593,588 | 1,514,759 | 1,451,081 | (142,507) | (8.9) |

Source: *Joint Annual Report of Hospitals, 1983-1985* (Memphis: Tennessee Health Resources Development Corporation, 1984-1986).

Med shows an almost 10 percent increase since 1983 while other area hospitals experienced a 9 percent drop. In August 1986, the Med's 499 available operational beds were fully occupied. Occupancy rates at other area hospitals were reported to be much lower.[25]

The statistics presented above indicate that the role the Med plays in providing health care in Shelby County is important and growing. The changes and improvements at the Med have come at a time when other area hospitals report financial pressures. Economic forces leading to unemployment and loss of health insurance, cutbacks in Medicare financing, and the saturation of the Memphis medical market have all served to sensitize the Med's competitors to the potential threat this hospital could represent.

Hospital administrators at competing institutions did not hesitate to state that the Med should remain an indigent care hospital. These officials were not supportive of the Med's attempts to become more like a private hospital and to shift some of the burden of uncompensated care to private hospitals. Some did not support the building of the new facility or the development of the trauma center. They stated that public hospitals should serve only public patients because of the tax support they receive. These individuals quite openly admitted to dumping indigent patients at the Med; they felt that their actions were justified by the large amounts of charity care they provided even though they felt under no obligation to provide this charity care.

Table 6.7

Gross Charges and Costs at
the Med and Other Area Hospitals, 1983

|  | Average Gross Charge per Inpatient Day | Average Cost per Inpatient Day |
|---|---|---|
| The Med | $635 | $529 |
| Baptist East | 822 | 365 |
| Methodist Central | 562 | 421 |
| UT/Bowld | 556 | 633 |
| St. Joseph's | 511 | NA |
| Baptist Memorial | 497 | 369 |
| Methodist South | 485 | 335 |
| Methodist North | 475 | 346 |
| Average for all nonfederal hospitals in Shelby County | $483 | $384 |

Source: *Data Supplement, 1983* (Memphis: Tennessee Health Resources Development Corporation, 1984).

NA: Not available.

A major stumbling block in the Med's becoming more competitive is its high costs and charges. As shown in Table 6.7, in 1983 the Med's charges were the second highest in Shelby County and its average cost per inpatient day was the highest. By 1986, costs had risen 16 percent, to $616 per inpatient day, and charges had gone up 44 percent, to $912 per inpatient day.[26] The Med will continue to be at a significant disadvantage in developing preferred provider or other alternative delivery system relationships with insurers or local employers if it does not bring its charges more into line with those of other area hospitals.

**Future Market Position of the Med**

The Med has witnessed significant changes in recent years, as evidenced by its change in governance, its increased emphasis on a more businesslike and efficient approach to operations, and its efforts to market itself as a higher-class hospital. The question remains as to how far it can evolve from its historical mission of serving the poor toward the private insurance payer model. The marketing strategies pursued by the Med's leadership play a significant part in determining its future role. At present, the hospital is faced with at least three choices concerning these strategies. Each choice has strengths and weaknesses, as well as different implications for efficiency of operations and access to care among the poor.

The first option is to continue to pursue its strategy of attracting more privately insured patients through marketing of the hospital's centers of excellence. This approach is likely to be continued, since early data suggest that the newly constructed facilities have had a positive effect on the Med's financial situation. Commercial revenues have grown and the number of patients treated in the Elvis Presley Trauma Center has been higher than expected: 700 patients were projected for 1984 and 1,160 were actually treated. Data from 1985 are even more positive. The trauma center treated over 1,600 patients, well over the projected volume of 850. In addition, total patient days at the hospital have increased as a result of the longer average length of stay for trauma center patients; emergency room visits have also increased.

Although these preliminary results look promising, questions remain. For example, detailed analyses have been performed to determine whether privately insured trauma center patients are being retained at the Med or are transferring out after they are stabilized. Detailed data on payer mix and patient origin for trauma center and emergency room patients are similarly lacking. The campaign to attract "Mr. and Mrs. Suburban" to the maternity service also has not been seriously evaluated. Moreover, efforts to market the Med's services to its own employees through a PPO arrangement have not been successful. Union officials viewed the plan as a "back-door approach to reduce the health care benefits of union members" and stated that management "can't force employees to use [the Med]."[27]

The hospital may face difficulties in further attempts to upgrade services or add specialized facilities. Unless completely subsidized by the county, the hospital will not be able to afford capital improvements. The Med is caught in the dilemma of needing to improve its physical plant to improve quality and attract privately insured patients while at the same time requiring revenues from such patients to improve its facilities. Because of the county's recent funding restrictions and the prospect of more severe cutbacks in the future, high levels of county support for capital improvements seem unlikely.

A second marketing strategy that the Med could use is to carve out a somewhat different market niche than the one described above. Instead of providing both a broad range of "low-tech" services to the poor and a set of "high-tech" services to commercially insured patients, the Med could try to occupy a more middle-of-the-road position. It could attempt to attract blue-collar, black and white citizens of Memphis who would use the hospital as their source of routine inpatient care. A key first step would be to attract more black physicians to the staff. Extending more admitting privileges to community physicians would also serve this goal.

Pursuing this market position would place the Med in direct competition with St. Joseph's, the Memphis hospital with the largest share of blue-collar patients and a large staff of black physicians. In such a competition, however, the Med might be in a strong position. If it can change the racial composition of its admitting staff, it may be able to use its strong teaching affiliation and centers-of-excellence image to penetrate the Memphis blue-collar market successfully. Efficiency may be enhanced by this strategy if these patients can be channeled into the large medical and surgical services, where occupancy rates are relatively low. Access for the poor would not be adversely affected, unless the Med was overwhelmingly successful in attracting working-class patients.

The third strategy for the Med is to become the center of an integrated county system of acute, ambulatory, and chronic care. Pursuit of this strategy would shift the Med's emphasis away from specialized services to primary and ambulatory care. Further, instead of seeking to attract privately insured patients, the hospital would focus on treating the indigent. Although the Med's administrators support such vertical integration and see more ambulatory care as the direction of the future, they are reluctant to give up the new high-tech, high-class, public hospital image. As one administrator put it: "The Med doesn't want to move completely back to primary care, but must have a marketing niche like neonatal intensive care."

There are many potential advantages in vertical integration for the Shelby County health care system. These include more emphasis on lower-cost ambulatory care; a decrease in inappropriate use of the emergency room through improved access to clinics and increased capacity at the public health clinics; better coordination with nursing homes, leading to more appropriate use of inpatient resources; and increased continuity and comprehensiveness of care through a shared medical staff. Efficiency would be improved by all these factors as well as by the ability to capture potential economies of scale. Access and quality of care for the indigent likewise would be improved.

By moving fully to this model, however, the Med would become completely dependent on the county for financial support. Many of the factors mentioned earlier may cause this to be an unwise choice. These include the erosion in the county's tax base, which necessitates funding limits, and the Med's lack of strong political backing at the state or county level. Even assuming that dramatic improvements in efficiency were possible, a complete move to a primary care, indigent facility model would be inadvisable. A more prudent course that would enhance fiscal viability would be to identify areas in which integration would be the least bureaucratically cumbersome. The hospital could move forward in these areas while maintaining and strengthening its marketing efforts toward privately insured patients.

## Summary

Before the governance change in 1980, Memphis' public hospital was besieged with problems: persistent and increasing operating losses; a lack of public credibility; lack of county support, including lack of agreement over whether a previously approved construction project should take place; and lack of a plan for funding projected operating expenses. In addition, it was widely felt that the needs of UT were being put before those of the poor and largely black community that the hospital was intended to serve.

The formation of the SCHCC in 1981 was credited with saving the hospital. Governance by the new entity increased community support by both whites and blacks and began to build the Med's reputation as a provider of high quality care to a potentially broad range of the residents of Shelby County. Although it is difficult to disentangle positive changes that occurred as a result of the new construction from the simultaneous governance change, evidence suggests that the county agreed to continue to fund the construction project because of the creation of SCHCC.

Although there have been some improvements in the hospital's finances as a result of the county-financed construction, the Med's operating deficit continues to be large. Financial problems that require increased attention include the contract to UT and low staff productivity.

While the continued existence of the Med is no longer in question as it was in 1980, the hospital's role as the area's major provider to the indigent requires it to rely on public support. The SCHCC has preserved the historical mission of the Med, perhaps at the price of not being able to become a hospital that competes successfully in the ever more competitive Memphis market for the privately insured. The Med's unit costs are high, and its image as Memphis's poor, black hospital is difficult to shed. The hospital faces the choice of continuing to try to become a high quality tertiary care hospital or seeking to become part of an integrated system of services for the indigent of Shelby County. The feasibility of the former course depends upon the county's willingness and ability to support past, current, and future construction efforts at the hospital. The attractiveness of the latter option depends upon the development of a rational, workable plan for sharing the costs of financing indigent care among area hospitals, local taxpayers, the business community, and state and federal programs.

## *Notes*

1. "Resource Inventory: The Regional Medical Center at Memphis, Memphis/Shelby County Health Department, Oakville and Shelby County Health Care Centers and Other" (Unpublished report of the Health Resources Development Corporation [HRDC], August 1986).
2. Unpublished data from HRDC.
3. Special tabulation from "Survey of Medical Care for the Poor and Hospitals' Financial Status, 1982" (Joint survey of the American Hospital Association and the Urban Institute).
4. Unpublished data supplied by the Regional Medical Center.
5. Ibid.
6. "Resource Inventory" (HRDC).
7. *Joint Annual Report of Hospitals, 1980-1985* (Memphis: Tennessee Health Resources Development Corporation, 1981-1986). There were 92,635 visits in fiscal year 1986, a 6 percent rise from 1985. This number is still well below the high of 170,277 reported in 1976.
8. Ibid.
9. Health Care Financing Administration, *Analysis of State Medicaid Program Characteristics* (Baltimore: U.S. Department of Health and Human Services, August 1985).
10. *Joint Annual Report* (HRDC).
11. "Resource Inventory" (HRDC).
12. Ibid.
13. Unpublished Regional Medical Center data.
14. Ibid.
15. "Resource Inventory" (HRDC).
16. Unpublished Regional Medical Center data.
17. "Resource Inventory" (HRDC).
18. Ibid.
19. Ibid.
20. Ibid.
21. Ibid., p. 50.
22. Unpublished Regional Medical Center data.
23. Ibid.
24. Ibid.
25. Unpublished data from HRDC.
26. Unpublished Regional Medical Center data.
27. "Union against Benefit Change," *Memphis Press-Scimitar*, 7 July 1983.

## ☙ 7 ❧

# Comparative Analysis of Efficiency and Access

## Kenneth E. Thorpe and Charles Brecher

This chapter provides a comparative analysis of the effect of two policy variables — governance arrangement and teaching commitment — on public hospital unit costs and on access to care by the urban poor. While several studies have attempted to assess the relative efficiency of public, private nonprofit, and for-profit institutions, there have been no major efforts to identify differences in efficiency among different types of public hospitals. Similarly, there are several studies describing the characteristics of hospitals providing relatively high volumes of care to the poor, but there have been no efforts to identify the contribution of public hospitals of different types to increasing access to care for the poor on a communitywide basis.

The two major sections of this chapter are devoted to the comparative analysis of efficiency and access. For both efficiency and access the sections present the hypothesized relationships with governance arrangements and teaching commitment, develop a statistical model to test the relationships, and summarize the results of the analysis.

### Efficiency

#### Hypothesized Relationships

For-profit hospitals generally seek to maximize profits, since profits provide income to the owners. One behavioral implication of profit maximization is cost minimization. Although not-for-profit hospitals may accumulate profits, they are not allowed to distribute the proceeds to trustees or boards of directors. Hence, a fundamental distinction in identifying the objectives of for-profit and not-for-profit firms is the extent to which the capitalized value of future profits is well defined. Since not-for-profit hospitals generally do not have well-defined residual claimants, their goals are more difficult to ascertain.[1] Because of the attenuation of property rights, not-for-profit hospitals are thought by some to be less efficient than for-profit hospitals.

While economic theory predicts that for-profit hospitals are more efficient than not-for-profit hospitals, few systematic predictions about efficiency among not-for-profit hospitals exist. Much of this ambiguity stems from the difficulty in determining the objectives of not-for-profit hospitals. These objectives have alternately been characterized as maximization of services, maximization of revenues, and maximization of a mix of services and quality. The observed objective of each hospital generally depends on the internal competition for resources among physicians, trustees, administrators, and others. Given the nature of this competition, the different theories of hospital behavior discussed in Chapter 2 provide only an ambiguous theoretical link between efficiency and ownership.

Despite the lack of agreement among theorists about the behavior of not-for-profit hospitals, public hospitals — particularly those operated as units of local government — are almost universally hypothesized to be less efficient than other hospitals. Rigidities inherent in local bureaucracies, budget maximization by bureaucratic decision makers, and the lack of property rights by any visible claimants (including salaried physicians) are expected to increase costs in public hospitals under direct government control.

Greater reliance on local tax subsidies may also affect the efficient operation of urban public hospitals. Although increased tax subsidies may add to the revenues of these hospitals, such increases may also reduce incentives for efficient operation.[2] The incentives to provide a given level and quality of hospital care at minimum cost may be reduced when local governments are the payer of last resort.

Larger teaching programs may also lead to greater unit costs. The hospital's teaching and research activities are commonly believed to generate higher indirect costs in the form of additional tests, hospital days, and ancillary services per discharge. Moreover, it is likely that physicians in teaching hospitals treat severely ill patients more aggressively than do physicians in other types of hospitals, and this also increases costs. These additional indirect costs are likely to increase with the size of a hospital's teaching program.[3]

## A Model for Analysis

An analysis of factors related to hospital efficiency requires the specification of a hospital cost function that relates to the cost of various inputs and the volume of output. Such a model should include an observable measure of cost to serve as the dependent variable, measures of each of the local policy variables, and measures of several control variables that should be taken into account to isolate the effects of the governance and teaching policies.

**Dependent Variable.** A cost function requires a standardized measure of hospital output. Since the ultimate output of a hospital — changes in health status — cannot be easily measured, some proxies are required. This analysis used hospital discharges as a measure of output. Admittedly, discharges are inexact measures because they do not recognize differences in the intensity of services provided in response to variations in patient treatment needs. They are, however, a better measure than most others — such as the number of inpatient days — because total discharges recognize variations in length of stay as well as in the volume of admissions. Moreover, as described below, variations in treatment needs can partly be recognized through existing controls for case mix.

Operating expenses per discharge are used as the measure of unit costs. Operating expenses are defined as total expenses less direct medical education costs and capital payments. This approach allows meaningful comparisons across teaching and nonteaching hospitals.

**Policy Variables.** The cost function estimation includes three policy variables of interest. Governance arrangements are included through dummy variables for each category (proprietary, voluntary, unit of local government, and semiautonomous public body). Dependence on local tax levy is measured as such revenue as a percentage of total expenses. The degree of teaching commitment is measured by the number of interns and residents per bed.

**Control Variables.** To assess accurately the effect of the three policy variables on interhospital differences in unit costs, it is necessary to control for other relevant variables. Among the most important of these control variables are the scale of the hospital's operations and the wages paid to employees. The number of inpatient beds and the wage per nonphysician, full-time-equivalent employee in each hospital are used as measures of these factors.

Another problem in estimating cost functions is to control for variations in the initial health status of the patients treated. This requires standardizing for variations in case mix among hospitals. A number of methods of standardizing for variations in cases treated have been suggested. To date, the only case mix measure available for most urban public hospitals is the diagnosis-related group measure used by the Medicare program. Although Medicare cases make up a relatively small proportion of the total case load of most public hospitals, the Medicare case mix index is correlated with other case mix measures for all hospital inpatients.[4]

Two other important control variables are the proportions of total hospital admissions covered by the Medicare and the Medicaid programs. These measures reflect differences in hospital costs that are due to variation in the severity of illness and to added fixed costs related to the treatment of low-income patients and that are not explicitly measured by the Medicare case mix index.[5]

Finally, the analysis includes the region in which a hospital is located, to take into account variations in physicians' practice patterns—such as differences in admitting patterns, lengths of stay, consultations and ancillary services—that vary regionally and are not otherwise reflected in the model.[6]

**Data Sources.** The two primary data sources for this analysis are the 1983 Annual Survey of Hospitals conducted by the American Hospital Association (AHA) and a 1983 survey of hospitals conducted jointly by the AHA and the Urban Institute. Although these surveys included a wider sample, we restricted our analysis to institutions in the 100 largest U.S. cities since our focus is urban public hospitals. Nearly 780 hospitals in the 100 largest cities provided enough data to be used in the analysis.

**Findings**

Application of the model described above to the available data provides insights into the character of local public hospitals in large cities as well as into the effects of the selected policy variables. Before presenting the results of the regression analysis, which isolates the effects of the selected policy variables, it would be useful to describe the characteristics of the large-city hospitals included in the analysis.

**Descriptive Statistics.** Local public hospitals are a minority of large-city hospitals (see Table 7.1). Public hospitals represent less than 7 percent of all large-city institutions; over three-quarters are voluntary hospitals and about one in six is a for-profit institution. The large-city

## Table 7.1

## Expenses per Discharge for Hospitals in 100 Largest U.S. Cities, 1982

| | *Percentage Distribution of Hospitals* | *Cost per Discharge*[a] |
|---|---|---|
| **Region** | | |
| New England | 2.7% | $4,027 |
| Middle Atlantic | 17.3 | 3,303 |
| South Atlantic | 11.9 | 2,804 |
| East North Central | 18.3 | 3,248 |
| East South Central | 8.0 | 2,152 |
| West North Central | 6.8 | 2,152 |
| West South Central | 14.6 | 2,350 |
| Mountain | 4.9 | 2,821 |
| Pacific | 15.5 | 3,405 |
| Total | 100.0% | $3,060 |
| **Governance** | | |
| Public—unit of local government | 3.6% | $4,426 |
| Public—separate board | 3.2 | 3,532 |
| Nonprofit | 75.5 | 3,112 |
| For-profit | 17.7 | 2,536 |
| Total[b] | 100.0% | $3,060 |

Sources: 1982 joint AHA–Urban Institute survey and 1983 AHA survey of hospitals.

Note: Data for 781 hospitals in survey supplying relevant data.

[a]Operating expenses exclusive of direct medical education and capital costs.

[b]Excludes state-owned public institutions.

hospitals—like large cities themselves—are unevenly distributed among regions of the nation. The East North Central states, the Middle Atlantic states, and the Pacific states have the largest share of hospitals; in contrast, the New England states have relatively few hospitals in large cities.

Average operating expenses per discharge vary widely by hospital governance structure—from a high of $4,426 in public hospitals controlled by a unit of local government to a low of $2,536 in for-profit hospitals. There also are significant differences in expenses per discharge between types of public hospital. Public hospitals with a semi-independent governing board have, on average, costs per discharge nearly $1,000 less than public hospitals operated as part of local government.

With respect to financing arrangements, most voluntary and proprietary hospitals receive no local subsidy (see Table 7.2). Among public hospitals, local subsidies averaged 7.8 percent of expenses, with a few public hospitals receiving no subsidy and some public hospitals covering more than 60 percent of their expenses with local subsidies. Teaching commitments also varied widely. The average large-city hospital had 6.3 interns and residents for every 100 beds, but the figures ranged from no teaching program to fully 70 interns and residents for every 100 beds.

Significant differences in hospital case mix and wage levels across governance structures were also evident. On average, the Medicare case mix was highest in public hospitals governed as a unit of local government and lowest in proprietary hospitals. Average case mix was approximately the same in semi-independent public and nonprofit hospitals.

The relationship between wages per nonphysician employee and governance revealed a different pattern; average nonphysician wages ranged from a high of $20,154 in nonprofit hospitals to a low of $18,303 in semi-independent public hospitals. Using the number of beds as an indicator of scale, public hospitals in the top 100 cities are considerably larger than other hospitals. The average number of beds in public hospitals exceeded 500—with semi-independent public hospitals topping the list at 534—compared to 381 and 174, respectively, in nonprofit and proprietary hospitals.

Finally, the payer mix differs across hospital types. Urban public hospitals provide care to larger proportions of Medicaid patients and relatively less care to Medicare patients than do other hospitals. These systematic differences in hospital payer mix and other control variables could account for some of the differences in unit costs among types of hospital.

In sum, the descriptive statistics paint an interesting picture of systematic differences in a number of important factors that influence cost per discharge. Most notably, urban public hospitals have higher operating costs, are larger teaching facilities, and have a more expensive mix of patients. They provide more service to Medicaid patients and less to patients covered under Medicare than do either proprietary or nonprofit hospitals. Average nonphysician wages are lower, on average, in public hospitals than elsewhere.

However, these simple cross tabulations may be misleading. The observed differences may be due to more complex relationships among the factors represented by the control and policy variables. To isolate the effect of governance structure, financing, and teaching commitment on operating costs requires multivariate analysis.

# Table 7.2
## Characteristics of Hospitals in 100 Largest Cities, 1982

| | All Hospitals (N = 781) | Public Hospitals Operated by Local Government (N = 18) | Public Hospitals Operated by Semi-independent Boards (N = 35) | Private, Nonprofit Hospitals (N = 590) | For-Profit Hospitals (N = 138) |
|---|---|---|---|---|---|
| Operating cost per discharge* | $3,060 | $4,426 | $3,532 | $3,112 | $2,536 |
| Medicare case mix index | 1.07 | 1.10 | 1.07 | 1.08 | 1.01 |
| Ratio of residents to beds | 0.06 | 0.18 | 0.14 | 0.07 | 0.00 |
| Medicare discharges as percentage of total | 30% | 18% | 18% | 31% | 31% |
| Medicaid discharges as percentage of total | 12% | 21% | 22% | 12% | 7% |
| Wage per nonphysician employee | $19,973 | $18,541 | $18,303 | $20,154 | $19,811 |
| Number of beds | 353 | 477 | 534 | 381 | 174 |
| Local government subsidy as percentage of expenses | 1% | 10% | 3% | 0% | 0% |

*Excludes capital costs and salaries of residents.

## Table 7.3

## Variables Used to Model Cost per Discharge, 1982
### (teaching hospitals)

| Variable | Regression Coefficient | Significance (p value) |
|---|---|---|
| Governance by unit of local government | 0.131 | <.10 |
| Governance by semiautonomous board | 0.175 | <.01 |
| Ratio of residents to beds | 0.099 | <.01 |
| Local government subsidy as percentage of expenses | 0.448 | .10 |
| Medicare case mix index | 0.917 | <.01 |
| Wages per nonphysician employee | 0.506 | <.01 |
| Number of beds | 0.017 | <.01 |
| Medicaid admissions as percentage of total | 0.079 | <.01 |
| Medicare admissions as percentage of total | 0.136 | <.01 |
| New England region | 0.223 | <.01 |
| Middle Atlantic region | 0.004 | .93 |
| South Atlantic region | (0.002) | .97 |
| East North Central region | 0.021 | .61 |
| East South Central region | (0.081) | .26 |
| West North Central region | (0.031) | .56 |
| West South Central region | 0.014 | .81 |
| Mountain region | (0.165) | <.05 |

Note: The constant for the equation is 3.506 and the adjusted $R$-square is 0.57. Pacific region is omitted and serves as a reference group.

**Regression Equation Results.** The model was tested using multivariate analysis in a log-linear (multiplicative) cost function. This functional form was selected because specification tests indicated that a log transformation of the dependent variable was approximately normally distributed. Normal plots indicated that a log-linear model yielded standardized residuals approximating a normal distribution.

The analysis was completed using available data for all hospitals in the 100 largest cities and separately using available data for all teaching hospitals in the 100 largest cities. The results from both analyses were highly consistent. Therefore, discussion will be focused on the results for teaching hospitals, where the findings are clearest (see Table 7.3). For reference purposes, the results of the analysis using data from all hospitals are presented in an appendix table.

After controlling for the relevant variables, operating costs per discharge in public hospitals are higher than in private hospitals. Costs per discharge in semi-independent public hospitals are over 19 percent higher, and costs in public hospitals operated as a unit of local government are nearly 14 percent higher, than costs in similar private hospitals. Between the two types of public hospital, there are no statistically significant differences in unit costs.[7] Thus, the particular form of public hospital governance does not have a significant influence on operating costs.

Teaching commitment does influence unit costs. Operating costs per discharge increase with the size of the graduate teaching program. Costs per discharge increase approximately $315 for each 10 percent increase in the ratio of interns and residents to beds. It should be noted that there is no discernible difference between public and private teaching hospitals in the added costs due to graduate medical education.[8]

With respect to financing arrangements, larger local tax levies do not appear to influence unit costs in public hospitals. Although the coefficient for the size of the local subsidy is quite large and positive, it is not statistically significant.

Operating costs increase with larger Medicare and Medicaid case loads, and the relationship does not differ across public and private hospitals. Specifically, operating costs per discharge increase approximately 1.9 percent for each 10 percent increase in the hospital's Medicare case load. Similarly, costs increase about 10 percent for each 8 percent increase in the Medicaid case load. These results are consistent with previous findings that costs are higher in hospitals serving a large or disproportionate share of low-income patients.

**Summary.** Three major findings emerge from the above analysis. Most important, there appears to be no statistically significant difference in unit costs between public hospitals with different governance arrangements. While the point estimates from the regression indicate that unit costs are approximately 5 percent higher among semi-independent public hospitals than among other public hospitals, the estimate is not statistically significant. Yet, after controlling for other relevant factors, urban public hospitals have higher costs than do similar private hospitals. Costs per discharge in urban public teaching hospitals are up to 20 percent higher than in urban private teaching hospitals.

Second, the results do not support the hypothesis that financing arrangements, specifically the extent of the local tax subsidies, affect unit costs. The relationship between the magnitude of local tax subsidy and the operating costs was large and positive, but not significant.

Third, even when controlling for case mix, larger graduate medical education programs were associated with increased costs per discharge. Costs increased approximately 1 percent for each 10 percent change in the ratio of residents to beds.

## *Access*

### Hypothesized Relationships

Previous research has established a strong relationship between hospital ownership and access to care by the poor.[9] These results indicate that urban hospitals, and in particular urban public hospitals, provide substantially more care to the poor than do other institutions. These studies also reveal that teaching hospitals provide a substantial volume of care to the poor. In some cases, teaching hospitals may rely heavily on charity care cases to provide material for clinical instruction and cases for research. In addition, the catchment areas of large teaching hospitals often include a significant volume of the poor. These results, therefore, are not especially surprising, given the concentration of the poor in urban areas as well as the traditional responsibility of the public hospital as the provider of last resort.

Existing differences among hospitals in the volume of care provided to the poor are likely to widen over time. Indeed, demand for care by the poor continues to climb as the growth in the population living at or just above the poverty line continues to increase. This population includes those of the poor who are eligible for Medicaid and/or Medicare as well as those without insurance. Although Medicaid was designed specifically to extend health insurance coverage to the poor, variations in state Medicaid eligibility requirements leave over one-half of the poor without health insurance coverage.[10] Often, the uninsured poor are employed by organizations that do not offer group health insurance programs, and they cannot afford to purchase individual insurance coverage. A growing body of research indicates that care for the poor — especially for those without insurance — is becoming more concentrated in public facilities as private hospitals become more reluctant to treat these patients.[11] Hospitals that traditionally covered care of the uninsured poor — much of it charity care — by increasing charges to charge-paying patients are also being squeezed. The growing reluctance of charge payers to finance a portion of charity care through hospital cost shifting, coupled with the continued decline in philanthropic contributions, may further reduce the incentive to provide care to the poor.

Although previous studies have supplied considerable information to policymakers documenting which hospitals provide care to the poor, there are still a number of unanswered questions. Most notably, what role do public hospitals in general, and their governance structures in particular, assume in increasing aggregate access to care by the poor? Further, do cities with large concentrations of graduate medical education in either public or private hospitals provide more care to the poor than do other cities? Examination of these questions requires a broader focus of inquiry, one that extends beyond individual hospitals. Specifically, is the total volume of care provided to the poor higher in communities with a public hospital system? Although public hospitals individually may provide a disproportionate share of care to the poor, their existence in any city may not increase overall access to care if private hospitals are less willing to accept poor patients. Moreover, there has been little previous work regarding the effect on access to care in cities that have "privatized" the public hospital system. Is access to care limited in these cities, or do private hospitals somehow pick up the slack?

The following sections present an empirical analysis of the effect of hospital governance and teaching intensity on care to the poor in a community. One specific hypothesis to be tested is that the volume of care provided to the poor in a community will be greater if the area has a public hospital, and will be greater in an area with a public hospital governed directly by a unit of local government rather than by a semi-autonomous board. That is, the governance structure of public hospitals is expected to influence provision of care to the poor. A public hospital with a semi-independent governance structure may be less politically accountable and place greater emphasis on the "bottom line" and less on its more traditional role as provider of last resort. A public hospital governed directly as a unit of local government may have the opposite organizational priorities.

A second hypothesis relates teaching commitment to the volume of care provided to the poor. For the reasons noted above, communities that have hospitals with larger teaching programs are expected to provide greater access to care for the poor in that community.

## Model for Analysis

Both descriptive and multivariate approaches will be used to analyze the effect of hospital governance structure and teaching intensity on access to care by the poor. The bivariate approach will evaluate the volume of care provided to the poor in four different types of cities: those with public hospitals governed as a unit of local government, those with public hospitals governed by a semi-independent board, those with state government hospitals, and those without any public hospital system. The average volume of care provided to the poor by hospitals in each ownership category will be examined within each city type.

For analysis, to isolate fully the effect of the two policy variables — governance structure and teaching commitment — on access to care by the poor, other relevant factors must be held constant. Indeed, utilization and supply of medical care depend on a variety of factors other than governance, ownership, and teaching. These control variables, as well as the measures of access, are discussed below.

**Dependent Variables.** Statistical analysis of this type requires an operational definition of access. There are at least two general methods of measuring access to care: process and outcome measures.[12] Process measures identify characteristics of the population at risk that could inhibit access to medical care. These measures include whether or not patients have a regular source of care, as well as factors known to affect health care utilization (such as travel and waiting time). Process measures are especially useful to evaluations when collected at the individual patient level, but less useful for the broader community focus of this study.

The second category of access measures includes outcome indicators that focus on the utilization of health care services by a defined population. A number of different outcome-based measures have been developed, varying with the service and population studied.[13] One especially useful outcome-based indicator of access is a measure of utilization by a defined population. For examining the volume of hospital-based (inpatient and outpatient) care to the poor, the following outcome-based measures are most relevant:

1. volume of uncompensated care adjusted admissions per poor uninsured population; and

2. volume of uncompensated and Medicaid adjusted admissions per poverty population.

Since the focus of this inquiry is local government hospitals and their primary catchment areas, the unit of measurement is the total volume — both inpatient and outpatient — of care provided in each city by all short-term general hospitals. This total volume is reflected in adjusted admissions, which convert outpatient visits to an appropriate volume of admissions.[14] The first measure relates uncompensated care to the uninsured poor; the second measure relates all care to the poor, including care to those with Medicaid coverage, to the area's poverty population.

The data used to measure the volume of uncompensated care are from a joint survey by the American Hospital Association and the Urban Institute.[15] Since it was difficult to discern the source of uncompensated care (i.e., inpatient versus outpatient), uncompensated charges were converted to equivalent uncompensated admissions by dividing uncompensated charges by the hospitalwide average charge per adjusted admission. However, a number of observations for uncompensated charges were missing from the data set. The missing data were estimated using a regression model that related uncompensated care admissions to the proportion of each hospital's Medicaid case load, the ratio of interns and residents to beds, the extent of city Medicaid coverage and hospital ownership, and the percent of cases admitted through the emergency room.

The analysis is restricted to the 100 largest cities in the United States. Although hospitals in the sample provide both inpatient and outpatient care to patients residing outside the city, the extent of border-crossing cases resulting in uncompensated care appears small. For example, in New York City, which has the largest city public hospital system, nonresident use of outpatient clinics accounts for less than 5 percent of all clinic visits. Moreover, inpatient admissions of residents from outside New York City account for less than 10 percent of all admissions. More important, the number of uninsured nonresidents (who are the primary recipients of inpatient uncompensated care) using New York City hospitals is minimal, accounting for less than 1 percent of all discharges.[16] While the evidence is not conclusive, the extent of such crossing apparently does not vary systematically across cities; therefore it should not appreciably alter the results of a comparative study. Nevertheless, to test for the importance of border crossing, a variable measuring the ratio of city population to county population was included in several regression equations. The results reported below were not affected by this broader market measure.

The 1982 uninsured poor population was calculated for each city based on the number of poor in the city (as estimated by the U.S. Census Bureau) minus the estimated number of Medicaid enrollees in the city. The estimate of Medicaid enrollees was based on the 1982 Medicaid eligibility level in the city's state. Specifically, the number of Medicaid enrollees in a city was estimated using the statewide ratio of

Medicaid enrollees to residents below the poverty line (as reported by the Health Care Financing Administration).

**Control Variables.** To isolate the effect of policy options for public hospital governance and teaching on access to care among the uninsured poor, analysis should consider other relevant factors. Previous research indicates that the supply of medical care to the poor, and their utilization of it, may vary with at least five factors: Medicaid coverage, minority population, elderly population, bed supply, and region.

Research examining the relationship between health insurance and utilization indicates that rates of hospitalization, ambulatory visits, and total expenditures vary with insurance status. For instance, expenditures for individuals with some health insurance who face high cost-sharing obligations are about 70 percent as high as expenditures for those receiving free care.[17] Thus, other factors constant, utilization—and hence access—will increase as the proportion of the poor with Medicaid coverage rises.

Because of complex eligibility requirements, which vary dramatically by state, Medicaid coverage for the poor is very uneven. These differences influence rates of utilization by the poor in different cities. Nationally, nearly one-half of those with incomes below the federal poverty level have Medicaid coverage, with the proportion varying from 17 percent in South Dakota to 104 percent in Hawaii.[18]

Numerous studies have discovered wide variations in hospital and ambulatory care use across racial groups within the same income category. Unadjusted use rates for black Medicaid enrollees are relatively low for almost all types of medical services.[19] Even after adjusting for demographic and health status differences, black Medicare enrollees have lower hospital admission rates than white enrollees.[20] Based on these and other similar findings, lower utilization rates are expected in cities with a larger nonwhite population. This control variable is measured as the proportion of the city's population that is nonwhite.

Most previous research indicates that the demand for and utilization of medical care among adults increases with age.[21] Hence, cities with a larger elderly population are expected to have higher utilization rates. This control variable is measured as the proportion of the city's population that is over age 65.

More than 25 years ago, Roemer raised the possibility that hospital use increases with the number and availability of hospital beds in an area.[22] A number of subsequent studies have found some evidence of the "Roemer effect." The estimated elasticity in these studies of per capita beds with respect to utilization has ranged from zero to over one.[23] Based on these results, the utilization-based access measure is expected to increase with the bed-to-population ratio in the community.

The region in which a city is located may also be an important control variable. Patterns of medical practice, including admission rates for the general population as well as for the poor, have been found to vary significantly among regions.[24] Four regional measures — East, West, South, and Midwest — were used in the analysis.

**Descriptive Statistics.** Table 7.4 displays the average volume of care to the uninsured poor as well as descriptive statistics for the policy variables and most of the control variables. Complete data were available for 99 of the 100 largest cities. Forty-eight of these cities had at least one local public hospital. Of cities with local public hospitals, 30 had public hospitals governed by semi-independent boards, while the public hospitals in 18 cities were governed as a unit of local government. Another 22 cities had no local public hospital but were the homes of state-sponsored public general hospitals which were typically operated by a state university system in conjunction with the university's medical school. Finally, another 29 cities had no public general hospital.

Cities with public hospitals had a greater concentration of teaching activity than other cities. Cities with semi-autonomous public hospitals had the highest average ratio of residents to beds; cities with state-run public hospitals were next highest, and cities without any public hospital had the least teaching activity.

Factors affecting the demand for care by the poor also varied widely across cities. The percentage of the poor covered by Medicaid ranged from a low of 39 percent in cities with semi-independent public systems to over 50 percent in cities with no public hospital. The racial composition of the cities also differed, with the minority population ranging from a low of 24 percent in cities without public hospitals to 37 percent in cities with semi-independent public hospital systems. The relative size of the elderly population was similar across all cities, however.

Supply conditions also varied among the cities. Average bed-to-population ratios were highest in cities without local public hospitals and lowest in cities with public hospitals governed as a unit of local government.

Because of the wide variation in underlying demand and supply characteristics, the volume of care to the poor differed across cities. On average, total (both uncompensated and Medicaid) utilization per

## Table 7.4

## Health System Characteristics in 100 Largest Cities, 1982
### (mean values)

| Variable | All Cities* (N = 99) | Cities With: | | | |
|---|---|---|---|---|---|
| | | Public Hospitals Unit of Local Government (N = 18) | Public Hospitals Semi-autonomous Boards (N = 30) | State-Run Public Hospitals (N = 22) | No Public Hospitals (N = 29) |
| Uncompensated and Medicaid adjusted admissions per poor population | 0.43 | 0.46 | 0.42 | 0.47 | 0.39 |
| Uncompensated care adjusted admissions per uninsured poor population | 0.30 | 0.34 | 0.31 | 0.34 | 0.24 |
| Ratio of residents to hospital beds | 0.085 | 0.089 | 0.102 | 0.091 | 0.064 |
| Percentage of poor covered by Medicaid | 44.5% | 48.9% | 39.0% | 39.9% | 50.6% |
| Minority share of population | 30.5% | 33.6% | 37.0% | 29.0% | 24.1% |
| Share of population over age 65 | 11.5% | 11.6% | 11.6% | 11.9% | 11.4% |
| Hospital beds per 1,000 population | 8.8 | 7.9 | 8.0 | 9.3 | 10.1 |

*Complete observations were not available for San Antonio.

## Table 7.5

### Estimated Mean Adjusted Admissions
### in 100 Largest Cities, 1982

| | Cities With: | | | |
|---|---|---|---|---|
| | *Public Hospitals Unit of Local Government* | *Public Hospitals Semi-autonomous Boards* | *State-Run Public Hospitals* | *No Public Hospitals* |
| Medicaid and uncompensated adjusted admissions[a] | 36,800 | 33,600 | 37,600 | 31,200 |
| Uncompensated adjusted admissions[b] | 15,096 | 13,764 | 15,096 | 10,656 |

[a]Estimated at mean poverty population size for the 100 cities.
[b]Estimated at mean uninsured poverty population size for the 100 cities.

poverty population was lowest in cities without public hospitals and highest in cities with state-run public hospitals. The relative volumes of care to the uninsured poor also differed across cities. Cities with state and local public hospitals provided a notably higher average volume of uncompensated care per uninsured poor person than did cities without public hospitals.

The significance of the magnitude of the differences in volume of care to the poor can be illustrated with figures indicating how the types of cities would differ on this measure of access if they all had the same number of poor residents (see Table 7.5). Assuming all cities had a poor population equal to the mean for the 100 largest cities, total (uncompensated and Medicaid) adjusted admissions of the poor would vary from a high of 37,600 in cities with state-run public hospitals to 31,200 in cities without public hospitals. Cities whose public hospitals are run as a unit of local government or by semiautonomous boards would provide, on average, 5,600 and 2,400 more adjusted admissions, respectively, than would cities without public facilities. Similar calculations for uncompensated care to the uninsured poor showed even greater differences. Cities with state-run hospitals and with hospitals operated as a unit of local government would provide over 4,400 more such uncompensated admissions than would those cities without public hospitals. Cities with public hospitals governed by semi-independent boards would provide over 3,000 (some 29 percent) more such uncompensated admissions than would cities without public facilities.

The presence of a public hospital not only increases the volume of care provided to the poor, it also reduces the uncompensated care burden for private hospitals. Uncompensated care averaged 5.9

percent of hospital charges in cities with no public hospital and 6.5 percent in cities with some type of public hospital. In cities with no public hospital, this financial burden was borne by private hospitals. In contrast, cities with a public hospital provided a greater total amount of uncompensated care and placed less financial burden on private hospitals. In these cities, private hospitals provided uncompensated care equal to just 4.4 percent of charges, while the public hospitals' much higher proportion (19.8 percent) raised the citywide average to 6.5 percent.

In summary, according to these bivariate comparisons, increased access to care by the uninsured poor in cities with public hospitals appears related to less care being provided to this population by private hospitals. At the same time, private hospitals in cities without a public hospital provide, on average, a greater volume of uncompensated care than do private hospitals in other cities.

Nevertheless, substantial variation across cities in underlying demand and supply characteristics could make the results implied by this bivariate analysis statistically insignificant and misleading. To account for these differences across cities and to isolate the effects of governance and teaching on access requires a multivariate approach. Accordingly, a multiple regression model was developed using the variables described above.

## Multivariate Analysis

A number of different model specifications were estimated. Finally, a model in a log-linear (multiplicative) form for the continuous variables was selected, because specification tests indicated that a log transformation of the dependent variable was approximately normally distributed. Moreover, normal probability plots indicated that a log-linear model yielded standardized residuals approximating a normal distribution. The model is displayed below:

$$\ln(\text{POOR}) = \alpha_0 + \alpha_1 (\text{LOC}) + \alpha_2 (\text{AUT}) + \alpha_3 (\text{STATE}) + \alpha_4 (\text{RES})$$
$$+ \alpha_5 \ln(\text{MIN}) + \alpha_6 \ln(\text{P65}) + \alpha_7 (\text{EAST}) + \alpha_8 (\text{SOUTH})$$
$$+ \alpha_9 (\text{MID}) + \alpha_{10} (\text{POP}) + e_t$$

where:

| | |
|---|---|
| POOR | = uncompensated care admissions equivalents/uninsured poor |
| LOC | = presence of a public hospital operated as a unit of local government |
| AUT | = presence of a public hospital operated under semiautonomous board |
| STATE | = presence of a public hospital operated by the state |
| RES | = city ratio of interns and residents to beds |

## Table 7.6

## Variables Used to Model Volume of Uncompensated
## Care to the Poor in 100 Largest Cities, 1982

| Variable | Regression Coefficient | Significance (p value) |
|---|---|---|
| Presence of public hospital operated as unit of local government | 0.397 | < .01 |
| Presence of public hospital operated under semi-autonomous board | 0.257 | < .05 |
| Presence of state hospital | 0.283 | < .05 |
| Ratio of residents to beds | 2.63 | < .01 |
| Percentage of population nonwhite | (0.204) | < .01 |
| Percentage of population over age 65 | (0.037) | 0.836 |
| Ratio of beds to population | 0.399 | < .01 |
| Location in East region | (0.422) | < .05 |
| Location in South region | (0.113) | 0.447 |
| Location in Midwest Region | (0.376) | < .01 |

Note: The constant is (.002) and the adjusted $R$-square is 0.242. All continuous variables are expressed in log form.

| MIN | = city percentage of nonwhite population |
|---|---|
| P65 | = city percentage of population over age 65 |
| EAST | = city located in East region |
| SOUTH | = city located in South region |
| MID | = city located in Midwest region |
| POP | = city ratio of population to beds |

Three dichotomous variables—public, unit of local government; public, semiautonomous board; and no public system—were used to indicate governance structure. Dichotomous variables were also used to indicate region, with the West serving as the reference region.

Uncompensated care for the uninsured poor was strongly influenced by the policy variables of governance structure and teaching commitment (see Table 7.6). Governance structure significantly influences the total amount of care provided to the poor. Most notably, cities with public hospitals provided more uncompensated care per uninsured poor person than other cities. The ratio of uncompensated adjusted admissions to uninsured poor was 40 percent higher in cities with public hospitals operated as a unit of local government than in cities without public hospitals. Cities with other types of public hospital governance also provided approximately 28 percent more uncompensated care per poor uninsured person than did cities without public hospitals.

The effect of a city's teaching commitment on communitywide levels of care provided to the uninsured poor is worth highlighting. The

## Table 7.7

## Variables Used to Model Total Volume of Care
## to the Poor in 100 Largest Cities, 1982

| Variable | Regression Coefficient | Significance (p value) |
|---|---|---|
| Presence of public hospital operated as unit of local government | (0.020) | .84 |
| Presence of public hospital operated under semi-autonomous board | 0.036 | .32 |
| Presence of state hospital | 0.022 | .23 |
| Ratio of residents to beds | 0.579 | .36 |
| Percentage of poor enrolled in Medicaid | 0.094 | < .05 |
| Percentage of population nonwhite | (0.147) | < .01 |
| Percentage of population over age 65 | (0.076) | .52 |
| Ratio of beds to population | 0.658 | < .01 |
| Location in East region | (0.265) | < .05 |
| Location in South region | (0.236) | < .05 |
| Location in Midwest region | (0.240) | < .05 |

Note: The constant is 1.635 and the adjusted $R$-square is 0.512. All continuous variables are expressed in log form.

regression analysis indicates that each 1 percent increase in the ratio of interns and residents to beds translates into a 2.6 percent increase in the ratio of uncompensated adjusted admissions to uninsured poor population. Hence, cities involved in a substantial volume of graduate medical education provide proportionately more care to the uninsured poor than do other cities.

Finally, the supply of beds in the community had a significant positive effect on uncompensated care, and the relative size of the minority population had a significant negative impact. The relative size of the aged population did not affect utilization. The regional variables for the East and Midwest indicate that these regions had significantly lower utilization than did the West, while the South was not significantly different from the West.

The regression equation for total (Medicaid and uncompensated) care provided to the poor indicated that neither of the policy variables, hospital governance and teaching commitment, was statistically significant (see Table 7.7). The principal factors explaining the volume of care provided to the poor in a community were the extent of Medicaid coverage, the relative size of the minority population, the local supply of hospital beds, and regional location.

More generous Medicaid coverage had a significant positive effect on access to care. According to the equation, a 10 percent increase in the proportion of the poor covered by Medicaid increased total admissions by 1 percent. Hence for the average-size city, if Medicaid coverage increased from 45 percent of the poor (the 100-city average) to 49 percent, total adjusted admissions would increase from 31,880 to 32,150.

The availability of beds in a city also had an important positive effect on utilization. The results indicate that a 10 percent increase in the bed-to-population ratio is associated with a 6.6 percent increase in utilization among the poor. Although the exact nature of this relationship continues to be debated, this finding is similar to findings in other studies that used different time periods and levels of aggregation.[25]

The size of a city's minority population, as hypothesized, had a negative influence on utilization. The equation indicates that a 10 percent increase in the minority proportion of the population translates into a 1.5 percent decrease in adjusted admissions among the poor.

Finally, the regional variables included to serve as proxies for omitted variables affecting utilization were significant. According to the results, utilization among the poor was between 27 percent and 30 percent lower in regions other than the West.

## Conclusion

This chapter has provided a unique comparative analysis of how policy decisions regarding governance structure and teaching commitment influence two important aspects of hospital system performance — efficiency and access. A regression model examined the relationships between these policy variables and efficiency to explain operating costs per discharge among all hospitals in the 100 largest cities; the factors affecting access were analyzed with a regression model explaining the volume of care to the poor and the volume of uncompensated care to the uninsured poor provided by all hospitals in each of the 100 largest cities.

With regard to efficiency, the analysis confirmed earlier findings that teaching programs significantly increase unit costs. While residency programs are widely believed to improve the quality of medical care, the price of such gains is substantial. This positive relationship between scale of teaching programs and unit costs was similar for private hospitals and public hospitals of all types.

The analysis also indicated that after controlling for all appropriate variables, public hospitals with semi-independent boards were not operated more efficiently than those run directly by a unit of local government. However, both types of public hospital had unit costs significantly higher than private hospitals, even after controlling for other related factors including case mix, teaching commitment, and local wage levels. The remaining cost differentials can be attributed to an unknown combination of differences in management styles, differences in quality, and unmeasured variations in severity of illness among patients served by each type of hospital.

With regard to access, the volume of uncompensated care provided to the uninsured poor in a city was strongly influenced by both the level of teaching activity and the presence of a public hospital. The greater the ratio of residents to beds, the greater the volume of uncompensated care provided in a city. Also, communities with public hospitals provided significantly more uncompensated care than did communities without public hospitals. There was no significant difference in the volume of uncompensated care between communities with public hospitals operated directly by local government and those with hospitals governed by semi-independent boards; both types were associated with higher levels of uncompensated care than was available in communities without public hospitals.

However, the total (Medicaid and uncompensated) volume of care provided to the poor in a community did not vary significantly with either the scale of teaching activity at the community's hospitals or the form of governance of the community's hospitals. The major factors explaining the total volume of care provided to the poor were the level of Medicaid coverage in the city, the overall bed supply in the community, and the relative size of the minority population.

The findings with regard to access suggest that voluntary hospitals, which constitute the vast majority of the nation's urban hospitals, are highly responsive to changes in the medical care financing system. When Medicaid coverage is relatively generous, private hospitals increase the volume of care they provide to the poor; when Medicaid coverage is more limited, they restrict such care.

Similarly, private hospitals appear to adjust their efforts to care for the uninsured poor depending on whether a local subsidy is available to finance a public hospital. In communities with a public hospital, the private institutions provide a lower volume of uncompensated care, and the public hospital accounts for a larger share of all uncompensated care and increases the citywide volume of such care. When no public hospital subsidy is available, private hospitals increase their uncompensated care but not by an amount sufficient to match the public hospital effort.

Overall, local sponsorship of a public hospital poses a trade-off. Whether operated by local government directly or by a semi-independent board, a public hospital appears to be a relatively expensive mechanism for delivery of care. However, the added local expenditures for such an institution do purchase a social good—an increment in access to care for the uninsured poor—that is not uniformly available from private institutions.

## Notes

1. See, for example, Harold Demsetz, "Some Aspects of Property Rights," *Journal of Law and Economics* 61 (April 1966): 1–22; and Louis De Alissi, "The Economics of Property Rights: A Review of the Evidence," *American Economic Review* 73, no. 1 (March 1983): 64–81.
2. Harvey Liebenstein, "Aspects of X—Efficiency of the Firm," *Bell Journal of Economics*, August 1975, pp. 580–606.
3. Frank Sloan, Roger Feldman, and Bruce Steinwald, "Effects of Teaching on Hospital Costs," *Journal of Health Economics* 2, no. 1 (1983): 1–28, and Kenneth Thorpe, "The Use of Regression Analysis to Determine Hospital Payment: The Case of Medicare's Indirect Teaching Adjustment," *Inquiry* 25, no. 2 (Summer 1988): 219–31.
4. Use of the Medicare case mix to characterize the case mix of all patients, especially in public hospitals, could be subject to measurement error. For instance, there is some concern that the current Medicare case mix index does not adequately reflect interhospital differences in the complexity or severity of patients treated. If, for example, public hospitals attract more complex patients than other hospitals, observed differences in costs—even after controlling for case mix using the Medicare index—may simply reflect unmeasured differences in complexity rather than inefficiencies. We used two approaches to reduce measurement error in the case mix index. The case mix index was "decompressed" by increasing the case mix index for more complex hospitals and reducing it for less complex ones. This factor, in part, corrects for severity differences currently not recognized in the Medicare case mix index. (See K. Thorpe, S. Cretin, and E. Keeler, "Are the DRG Weights Compressed?" *Health Care Financing Review*, forthcoming.) Second, we included the proportion of public patients treated by the hospital. Inclusion of these variables recognizes and partially accounts for unmeasured differences in patient complexity within the current Medicare case mix indexes. Moreover, use of these additional case mix proxies recognized the limitations of using a scalar measure of hospital case mix in any cost function. Finally, unpublished calculations by the author using New York data indicate that the correlation between the Medicare case mix index and one constructed for all patients exceeds .7.
5. Kenneth E. Thorpe, "Why are Urban Hospital Costs So High? The Relative Importance of Patient Source of Admission, Teaching, Competition, and Case Mix," *Health Services Research* 22, no. 6 (February 1988): 821–36.
6. D. L. Rothberg, ed., *Regional Variations in Hospital Use* (Lexington, MA: D.C. Heath and Company, 1982).
7. For the interpretation of dummy variables in semilog equations, see Peter Kennedy, "Estimation with Correctly Interpreted Dummy Variables in

Semilogarithmic Equations," *American Economic Review* 71, no. 4 (September 1981): 801.

8. This conclusion is based on a variation of the regression equation summarized in Table 7.3, which also included variables representing the interaction of governance variables and the ratio of residents to beds. These variables did not have statistically significant coefficients.

9. Judith Feder, Jack Hadley, and Ross Mullner, "Falling Through the Cracks: Poverty, Insurance Coverage, and Hospital Care to the Poor, 1980 and 1982," *Milbank Memorial Fund Quarterly* 62, no. 4 (Fall 1984): 544–66; Frank Sloan, Joseph Valvona, and Ross Mullner, "Identifying the Issues: A Statistical Profile," in Frank Sloan, Joseph Valvona, and Ross Mullner, eds., *Uncompensated Hospital Care, Rights and Responsibilities* (Baltimore: Johns Hopkins University Press, 1986); and Kenneth E. Thorpe and Charles Brecher, "Improved Access to Care for the Uninsured Poor in Large Cities: Do Public Hospitals Make a Difference?" *Journal of Health Politics, Policy and Law* 12, no. 2 (Summer 1987): 313–24.

10. Health Care Financing Administration, *Characteristics of State Medicaid Programs, 1984* (Baltimore: U.S. Department of Health and Human Services, 1986).

11. See, for example, Robert Schiff et al., "Transfers to a Public Hospital: A Prospective Study of 467 Patients," *New England Journal of Medicine* 314, no. 9 (17 February 1986): 552–57; and "Hospitals in Cost Squeeze 'Dump' More Patients Who Can't Pay Bills," *Wall Street Journal*, 8 March 1985.

12. Access to care can be characterized by a number of indicators including measures of *potential* as well as *actual* utilization of services. For a discussion of access measures, see Lu Ann Aday and Ronald Andersen, *Development of Indices of Access to Medical Care* (Ann Arbor, MI: Health Administration Press, 1975).

13. Ibid.

14. The formula for adjusted admissions is:

$$\text{Adjusted admissions} = \text{admissions} \times \frac{\text{total revenue}}{\text{inpatient revenue}}$$

15. The data set used is the joint survey of the American Hospital Association and the Urban Institute, "Survey of Medical Care for the Poor and Hospitals' Financial Status, 1982." It contained information on uncompensated care charges. To make these data comparable to data on the volume of Medicaid services, we converted uncompensated charges to equivalent uncompensated admissions by dividing uncompensated charges by total charges for all care over total admissions. Medicaid outpatient visits were converted to admissions by dividing these visits by the product of three times the average length of stay. This methodology is similar to that used by the American Hospital Association to calculate adjusted admissions.

The data set also was missing a number of observations for hospital Medicaid outpatient visits and for uncompensated care charges. To complete the analysis, however, observations on all hospitals in the 100 largest cities were required. Missing data on uncompensated care were estimated using a regression model relating uncompensated care admissions to the proportion of each hospital's Medicaid case load, the ratio of interns and residents to beds, and the extent of city Medicaid coverage. Since most of the missing data were for urban private hospitals, the regression excluded public hospital data. Missing Medicaid outpatient visits were estimated using each city's ratio of Medicaid inpatient to outpatient visits.

Finally, the relevant market for the analysis was restricted to hospitals in the 100 largest cities. Although previous research indicates a substantial volume of border crossing of patients across city, county, and state lines to receive medical care, such crossing is probably minimal in the case of the poor. Nevertheless, to test for the possibility of border crossing, a variable measuring the ratio of city population to county population was included in several regression equations. The results reported below were not affected by this broader market measure. For a discussion of the importance of patient border crossing, see Miron Stano, "An Analysis of the Evidence on Competition in the Physician Services Markets," *Journal of Health Economics* 4, no. 3 (September 1985): 197–211; and Joseph P. Newhouse et al., "Where Have All the Doctors Gone?" *Journal of the American Medical Association* 247 (1982): 2392–96.

16. *Inpatient Hospital Use in New York City, 1982* (New York: United Hospital Fund, 1983); and *Ambulatory Care in New York City, 1984: Patient Characteristics and Patterns of Hospital Use* (New York: United Hospital Fund, 1984).
17. J. P. Newhouse et al., *Some Interim Results from a Controlled Trial of Cost Sharing in Health Insurance*, R-2847-HHS (Santa Monica, CA: Rand Corporation, January 1982).
18. Health Care Financing Administration, *The Medicare and Medicaid Data Book, 1984* (Baltimore: U.S. Department of Health and Human Services, 1986), Tables 1.1, 1.2.
19. Ibid.
20. M. Ruther, "Medicare: Use of Short Stay Hospitals by Aged and Disabled Inpatients, 1978," in *Health Care Financing Program Statistics* (Washington, DC: U.S. Government Printing Office, 1983); and Office of Statistics and Data Management, *Medicare Statistics*, HCFA Publication no. 03189 (Washington, DC: U.S. Government Printing Office, December 1984).
21. This literature is reviewed in L. A. Aday, R. Andersen, and G. V. Fleming, *Health Care in the U.S.: Equitable for Whom?* (Beverly Hills, CA: Sage Publications, 1980).
22. M. Roemer, "The Supply of Beds: A Natural Experiment," *Hospitals* 35 (1961): 35–42.
23. P. Ginsburg and D. Koretz, "Bed Availability and Hospital Utilization: Estimates of the Roemer Effect," *Health Care Financing Review* 5 (1983): 87–92.
24. D. L. Rothberg, *Regional Variations in Hospital Use.*
25. These studies are summarized in Ginsburg and Koretz, "Bed Availability and Hospital Utilization."

## Appendix Table

## Variables Used to Model Cost per Discharge, 1982
## (all urban hospitals)

| Variable | Regression Coefficient | Significance (p value) |
|---|---|---|
| Governance by unit of local government | 0.260 | <.01 |
| Governance by semi-autonomous board | 0.201 | <.01 |
| Ratio of residents to beds | (0.340) | <.01 |
| Local subsidy as percentage of expenditures | 0.043 | .12 |
| Medicare case mix index | 0.833 | <.01 |
| Wages per nonphysician employee | 0.421 | <.01 |
| Number of beds | 0.020 | <.05 |
| Medicaid admissions as percentage of total | 0.046 | <.01 |
| Medicare admissions as percentage of total | 0.140 | <.01 |
| New England region | 0.138 | <.05 |
| Middle Atlantic region | (0.029) | .35 |
| South Atlantic region | (0.061) | <.10 |
| East North Central region | 0.009 | .77 |
| East South Central region | (0.179) | <.01 |
| West North Central region | (0.008) | .85 |
| West South Central region | (0.073) | <.05 |
| Mountain region | (0.179) | <.01 |

Note: The constant for the equation is 4.237 and the adjusted $R$-square is 0.53. Pacific region is omitted and serves as a reference group.

# ᘒ 8 ᘓ

# Conclusion: Improving Public Hospital Performance

## Stuart H. Altman and Charles Brecher

The case studies and comparative analyses presented in this book suggest that policy decisions can improve the performance of urban public hospitals, but that there is no magic solution that will free city or county governments from their responsibilities to finance the hospital care of their indigent or poorly insured populations. This absence of a simple solution is particularly important today because public hospitals in general, and urban public hospitals in particular, face a growing set of problems. The combination of limited public funds and the increase in price competition throughout the U.S. health care system has put public institutions in an anomalous situation. Their role as the medical care system of last resort for the uninsured and the indigent has never been more critical. But many public institutions increasingly lack the financial capacity to provide this care at acceptable levels of quality and at a cost that governments can afford.

State and local officials have tried to influence the performance of their city or county health systems by restructuring the hospitals' governance structures, improving and restructuring their financial capacities, or revising their medical staff arrangements. But many of the easy solutions suggested to deal with the problems of public hospitals do not seem to work. To understand the interconnectedness of these issues and the workings of public hospitals, the public hospital systems in four urban areas—Los Angeles, Memphis, New York City, and Tampa—

were analyzed. In addition, information on the provision of hospital care to low-income populations in 100 of the largest urban areas in the United States was collected and analyzed. Three criteria were used to assess the performance of these public hospital systems: the degree of access afforded the indigent, the quality of services provided, and the efficiency of the provision of services. These three standards offer a basis for organizing the general lessons distilled from this volume.

## *Access*

The primary mission of hospitals established by cities and urban counties is to provide care to residents regardless of their ability to pay. Numerous studies document the large volume and disproportionate share of care to the indigent rendered in urban public hospitals. For example, a comprehensive survey in 1982 revealed that in the nation's 100 largest cities, local public hospitals represented only 10 percent of the hospital beds but accounted for fully 50 percent of the bad debt and charity care and 22 percent of the Medicaid care. No new evidence is needed to affirm the large role urban public hospitals play in caring for the poor.

However, elected officials often are concerned about the effectiveness of public hospitals in assuring access for the poor and in providing needed services efficiently. Some believe that private, usually nonprofit, hospitals in the community are capable of caring for the indigent and would do so if a public facility were not available. These critics suggest that local government subsidies to public hospitals are an ineffective use of taxpayers' money. A counterargument is that health care for the indigent is not free regardless of where it is provided. In cities with no public institutions, care in community hospitals is paid for either directly by the local government or indirectly through a hidden tax on the bills of privately insured patients treated in those institutions. The issue is, therefore, determining which system is more efficient and whether the community hospitals can effectively fulfill this public responsibility.

The data presented in Chapter 7 indicate that private hospitals do provide relatively more care for the poor in cities without public hospitals than do private hospitals in cities with public hospitals. However, the total care provided to these population groups in cities without public institutions is lower. In cities without a public hospital, private institutions devoted 5.9 percent of their revenues to uncompensated care, while the share was just 4.5 percent in cities with a local public hospital. But this is only half the story. The additional effort of voluntary institutions in the absence of a public hospital does not fully replace the indigent care available at public facilities. In cities without a public hospital—despite the higher levels of uncompensated care by voluntary institutions—the total volume of care provided to the uninsured poor is less than in cities with a public hospital. The increased access due to the presence of a public hospital is substantial; uncompensated care represented fully 6.5 percent of all hospital revenues in communities with a public hospital, compared to 5.9 percent in other areas. For a typical city among the nation's 100 largest, this translates into more than 31,000 additional uncompensated admissions annually due to the presence of a public hospital.

These figures suggest that decisions about the sponsorship and financing of urban public hospitals reflect political judgments not just about who shall pay for that care but also about how much care will be available to the uninsured poor. In the absence of a public hospital, voluntary hospitals are likely to provide some access to care for the poor and to finance that care with some combination of cost shifting and philanthropy. But a tax subsidy to a local public hospital does more than replace this private effort. Tax support for public hospitals buys a social good in the form of additional care for the uninsured poor.

Although urban public hospitals typically play a large and irreplaceable role in caring for the poor, the case studies reveal that they modify this commitment during certain periods. The Hillsborough County Hospital Authority (HCHA) in Tampa is an example of a public system that reduced its care to the poor significantly. Between 1982 and 1984 HCHA discharges dropped 16 percent and ambulatory visits fell 40 percent, largely as a result of policy decisions intended to curb services to Medicaid and uninsured patients. In contrast, the hospitals operated by the Los Angeles County Department of Health Services increased their admissions 18 percent and their ambulatory care visits 19 percent in a two-year period. Virtually all the additional care provided to medically indigent adults shifted from the state of California's Medicaid program to county responsibility. In this instance, LA County also received a sizable infusion of state funds to pay for these new patients.

Why do public hospitals change their levels of service to the poor in their communities? The answer seems to be a combination of money and politics. Money—that is, changed patterns of hospital financing—is not by itself a sufficient explanation of changes in commitment to care for the poor. Consider the contrasting examples of the HCHA and the New York City Health and Hospitals Corporation (HHC). In the period following New York City's fiscal crisis of 1975, the HHC had its local tax subsidy reduced and its Medicaid revenues tightly regulated.

Despite rapid inflation in the period from 1975 to 1980, its budget remained nearly frozen. Yet HHC maintained its volume of services and continued to provide care at the same level to indigent New Yorkers. In contrast, when Hillsborough County reduced its appropriation to HCHA and the state of Florida imposed caps on Medicaid outpatient payments, the HCHA board responded by sharply curtailing services to the indigent.

The HHC and HCHA examples are also illuminating because each of these hospital systems is governed by a semiautonomous board rather than operated directly by a unit of local government. The contrasting outcomes under seemingly similar governance structures suggest that one must look beyond legalities to political realities to understand the access policies of local public hospitals. In New York the "autonomous" board does not function with any significant political autonomy but remains closely allied with the mayor and his administration; in Tampa the creation of the HCHA was only one step in a political strategy to reduce the county's attachment to the public hospitals and to the general mission of personal health care. Thus, in Tampa a combination of reduced political and financial support from the county underlay the access restrictions; in New York continued political commitment to serving as a provider of last resort meant other types of adjustments were made when resources were constrained.

Money and politics interacted differently in Los Angeles to cause the Los Angeles County Department of Health Services to increase significantly its care to the county's indigent. As a unit of local government the LA system is closely supervised by elected county officials. Historically, a high level of access has been maintained in the county hospitals, partly because of community advocacy efforts. When the state transferred responsibility for medically indigent adults (MIAs) from its Medi-Cal program to county governments and earmarked additional financial resources to help the counties, the political leadership of LA took on an expanded role. Political will, backed by additional funds, led to expanded services for the poor at county facilities. Although state policies limited the choice of providers for the MIAs, county actions helped maintain the availability of needed care. Although the transfer was a clear-cut financial advantage to the county in the first year of the program, later cuts in state funds, plus increased patient demands, have put into question whether this program is really a fiscal benefit to LA County in the long run. Although the county continues to seek to provide all medical indigents with the medical care they require, the limited state funding and revised Medi-Cal policies have led to access difficulty for the MIAs.

The case studies also underscore an important point about the financing of urban public hospitals. The distinguishing feature of these hospitals is not just their access to local tax subsidies; they also rely heavily on state appropriations in the form of Medicaid revenues. Although Medicaid accounts for only 11 percent of hospital revenues nationwide, among urban public hospitals revenues from Medicaid average about one-fifth of total revenues, compared to an average 24 percent of revenues coming from local tax subsidies. In each of the four case study systems, Medicaid revenues were actually greater than local government subsidies. Medicaid policies also play an important role in determining the extent to which private hospitals in a city will provide care to the poor. Where provider payment rates and client eligibility are more generous, the private sector will provide more indigent care. Thus the finances of urban public hospitals and their capacity to provide indigent care are often shaped as much by state policies as by the decisions of local governments.

Events in Los Angeles dramatically illustrate this point. The decision of the state of California to shift the medical care responsibility for all MIA patients to the counties and to provide counties with most of the funds previously spent on these patients represented an important shift in the public financing of indigent patient care. Although the state was motivated in part by the desire to curb its budget growth, it also was encouraged to introduce this change to bolster the shaky financial position of most county public hospitals. Since the initial shift of responsibility, much effort has gone into debating the appropriate state funding level for these patients. What should not be missed, however, are the underlying philosophical goal of the program and its implications for the future funding of public hospitals and the care of the indigent.

The theme of the 1965 Medicare and Medicaid programs was that the aged and poor should have access to the mainstream of American medicine. No longer would these patients have to seek care at public institutions or be treated as charity patients at private or community hospitals. Most of the new programs of the 1970s followed that theme. Yet the need for public hospitals in most regions was not eliminated. Quite the contrary — a large proportion of the poor and aged continued to rely upon these public institutions as their medical care providers. With state and local medical care funds dispersed throughout the total health system, most public hospital systems continued to suffer from inadequate financial resources. The California MIA transfer program represents a direct means of rechanneling some of the public monies into these public institutions. It is an approach that has not been adequately evaluated, but it could become a model for other states, particularly if reasonably funded.

A final point about the commitment of urban public hospitals to ensuring access is that medical staffing policies influence the volume of care provided to the poor. The statistical analysis in Chapter 7 revealed, after controlling for other factors, that cities whose hospitals engage in a greater level of teaching activity provide a higher volume of uncompensated care to the uninsured poor. Among the four case study systems, the HCHA was the only public system with relatively weak teaching affiliations, and HCHA most readily reduced services to the poor when faced with fiscal constraints. Conversely, physicians at affiliated teaching institutions sometimes serve as advocates for indigent care. This was evident in Los Angeles and New York City. Thus, close alliances with major teaching institutions appear to reinforce other local policies that lead to a commitment to providing needed service to the indigent.

## Quality

Gauging the quality of medical care is a complex task, but the criteria established by the Joint Commission on the Accreditation of Healthcare Organizations are widely viewed as a basis for defining minimum acceptable standards. By these standards, urban public hospitals provide care of acceptable, and often of competitive, quality. In each of the case studies, the public facilities were granted Joint Commission accreditation, and any deficiencies cited did not relate to clinical care standards. A separate study conducted in New York City found that the HHC facilities had fewer deficiences in some areas than voluntary hospitals of similar size in that city.

However, one critical component of the quality of hospital care appears to be low for public institutions—the staffing levels of skilled nursing personnel. In New York City a special study revealed serious gaps between levels of public hospital nurse staffing and the standards suggested by the state hospital association. In other case studies, the public hospitals had fewer registered nurses relative to their work load than did regional and national comparison groups. This shortage of skilled nurses exists despite overall staff-to-work-load ratios that are high relative to other hospitals. The extent to which the distinct staffing patterns of public hospitals affect the quality of nursing care is not easily measured, but many view those staffing patterns as an indicator of lower quality care provided in these institutions.

The weaknesses of urban public hospitals and their reputations in some quarters for low quality also appear to be related to the status of their physical plants. Local governments tend to let their hospitals function without major rehabilitation or reconstruction for relatively long time periods, and this results in public perceptions of poorer hospitals with older facilities. This was widely reported to be the case in Los Angeles, and the lack of capital investment in New York City since the early 1970s created similar problems for some of its facilities. In contrast, the new construction efforts in Tampa and Memphis are widely perceived as measures that improved quality at the public hospitals. In the public's eye, physical appearance is equated with quality; limited capital investments by the public sector reinforce the image of urban public hospitals as second-class institutions.

In this sense, quality of care — or, more accurately, perceived quality of care — is affected by governance policies. Because public perceptions of quality are strongly related to hospitals' physical condition, access to capital for renovation and reconstruction has an important influence on perceptions of quality. Governance changes in the form of newly established public benefit corporations led to major capital investments in both Tampa and Memphis, because the new entities could issue revenue bonds independent of the local general government. In contrast, the Los Angeles public hospital system remains part of a fiscally pressed county government that has been unable to issue bonds because of tax limitation measures; consequently, its physical plant has not been renewed and its image suffers.

Finally, the case studies suggest that it is not universally true that medical school affiliations are essential for assuring quality medical care at a public hospital. In Tampa, there is a relatively weak affiliation, but the hospital maintains competitive quality standards. Two of the 11 acute care hospitals in New York City (Woodhull and Coney Island) have no contractual affiliation with an academic institution, and their quality does not seem to suffer. As the supply of physicians nationally has grown, there is growing flexibility for public hospitals to devise new medical staffing patterns.

Despite the greater availability of physicians, as well as positive steps such as gaining independent access to capital markets, public hospitals still face difficulty in becoming institutions that successfully compete with private community hospitals for insured middle-class patients. In the two case study sites where major efforts were made to alter market positions in this way, the results are at best uncertain. In Memphis, the construction of a new trauma center and significant marketing efforts did not yield a meaningful change in the economic mix of the patient population. In Tampa, the prospects for change as a result of the new facilities and favorable publicity are greater, but the hospital began with an unusually high share of privately insured patients; the long-run ability of the HCHA to improve its position in the very competitive local market remains uncertain.

## Efficiency

The comparative statistical analysis indicates that urban public hospitals have significantly higher costs per admission than their private counterparts. This remains true even after adjustments are made for several relevant factors, including the case mix of patients served and the local area wage scales. Furthermore, it is true both for public hospitals operated directly by local governments and for those operated by semiautonomous boards. Thus, where the analysis indicates less efficient operations at public hospitals, the difference persists even when efforts are made to establish a more politically autonomous governance structure.

Of course, the difference in costs per admission between public and other hospitals should not automatically be assumed to be a matter of inefficient management. All relevant factors cannot be adequately incorporated into the statistical analysis, and some of the difference may be attributed to such unmeasurable factors as the social service needs of the poorest patients and the severity of illness of patients that is not captured in available case mix indices. The case studies do point, however, to some seemingly inefficient management practices. Each of the case studies revealed higher staff-to-work-load ratios at public hospitals than at relevant comparison groups of hospitals. Yet this was not the case for all types of personnel. As noted earlier, registered nurses are underrepresented at public hospitals, and most of the additional staff are less-skilled support personnel. This, rather than excessive wage levels, is apparently the major contributor to higher than expected unit costs. Such evidence is consistent with frequently voiced views that public hospitals tend to serve as a source of employment in lower-income communities and thereby serve a political function.

The analysis of efficiency at urban public hospitals is enriched by the case studies, which demonstrate that it is possible for these institutions to improve their efficiency markedly in a relatively short time. The New York City HHC, the Tampa HCHA, and the Los Angeles DHS each achieved notable improvements in their relative efficiency during the case study period. Unit costs at these institutions, while remaining high, fell relative to their peer groups during the early 1980s.

The ways these gains in relative efficiency have been achieved differ from the policy prescriptions often urged on public officials. The theoretical benefits of independent governance and associated businesslike practices were not evident. In fact, in each of the three cities that established independent boards, expenditures and unit costs grew rapidly in the period after the board's creation. The gains in efficiency occurred when resources were constrained; that is, fiscal problems improved efficiency. In New York City, the local government's fiscal crisis limited appropriations to the HHC; the agency maintained its service commitment by slowing the pace of wage increases and operating with a reduced complement of staff. Similarly, the 1983 fiscal crisis for the HCHA led to staff reductions and slowed budget growth, which lowered relative unit costs. In Los Angeles, where an independent board has not been established, significant efficiency gains followed the large utilization increases that resulted from the shift of responsibility for MIAs from the state to the county. Faced with a substantial increase in its service volume and a disproportionately small increase in its budget, the DHS devised ways to meet its clients' needs despite constrained resources.

In brief, fiscal stringency, rather than planned structural reforms, served as the principal stimulus for greater efficiency. But a caveat must be offered with this conclusion. An important unknown in each of the case studies is the extent to which the efficiency gains also represent reductions in quality of care. Although there were no reports of generally substandard care during any of the periods of fiscal stringency, the public hospitals have retained their reputations as second-class institutions. Part of the explanation may be the seemingly inefficient mix of labor and capital and the combination of overutilization of less-skilled personnel and underutilization of more-skilled nurses. But other factors are also at work. American society is both ideologically biased in favor of private institutions and racially biased against minority groups. Consequently, public institutions serving a predominantly poor and ethnically mixed clientele may be labeled by the white middle class as inferior in quality regardless of more objective evidence.

## Summary

Overall, the evidence assembled in this book indicates there is no quick fix for the problems faced by urban public hospitals. These institutions are capable of expanding access to care for their community's indigent residents, of providing care to these and other residents that is of acceptable quality and comparable to that of private institutions, and of improving their relative efficiency to bring their unit costs more in line with similar private institutions. But achieving these goals is not simply a matter of changing the formal structure of governance or altering affiliation arrangements with academic institutions. Urban public hospitals remain strongly attached to their local political structures under virtually all circumstances. Consequently, the most important factor influencing the financial strength of these institutions as well as the quality of care they provide is the fiscal condition of their state and local governments combined with the social philosophy of their community toward their public hospital system.

However, even the right combination of political will and financial resources may not be sufficient to reverse rapidly the long-standing public prejudices against using public facilities when private institutions are available. Therefore, successful operation of a public institution requires a close link with the dominant political system in the area. State and federal governments also should bear in mind that changes in their reimbursement policies for Medicaid have a disproportionate effect on public hospital systems. Under such conditions, citizens' expectations for local public hospitals should reflect a balanced understanding of both the possible achievements and the obstacles to reaching them.

# Index

# About the Editors

STUART H. ALTMAN is Dean of the Heller Graduate School for Social Policy, Brandeis University, and Sol C. Chaikin Professor of National Health Policy. He is in his second term as Chairman of the congressionally legislated Prospective Payment Assessment Commission, which is responsible for overseeing the Medicare DRG Hospital Payment System. Between 1971 and 1976, Dean Altman was Deputy Assistant Secretary for Planning and Evaluation/Health at the Department of Health, Education, and Welfare. While serving in that position, he was one of the principal contributors to the development and advancement of the administration's national health insurance proposal. From 1973 to 1974, he served as Deputy Director for Health of the President's Cost-of-Living Council where he was responsible for developing the council's program on health care cost containment. He has a Ph.D. in Economics from the University of California, Los Angeles and has taught at Brown University and University of California, Berkeley.

CHARLES BRECHER is Research Director for the Citizens Budget Commission in New York and Professor at the Graduate School of Public Administration, New York University. He is also codirector of the Setting Municipal Priorities project at New York University with Columbia University, and is principal investigator of a series of funded research projects for the Graduate School of Public Administration, New York University. He has served as a consultant for a number of corporate and public studies and research programs and has written numerous books and articles. He has taught at the New School for Social Research, Columbia University, and Fordham University. Dr. Brecher holds a Ph.D. in Political Science from the Graduate Division of the City University of New York.

MARY G. HENDERSON is a Senior Research Associate and Adjunct Lecturer at the Bigel Institute for Health Policy Studies, Heller School, Brandeis University. Her primary research interest is the evaluation of managed care plans for high-cost and at-risk populations. She works extensively with state governments, large employers, and federal agencies to design, implement, and evaluate managed care initiatives. Previous research projects include the study of inpatient and ambulatory patient classification systems and physician payment issues. She is a member of the Association for Health Services Research and the American Public Health Association. Dr. Henderson received her Ph.D. in Social Policy at the Heller School, Brandeis University.

KENNETH E. THORPE is an Assistant Professor of Health Economics in the Department of Health Policy and Management, Harvard School of Public Health. He has also served as consultant to the Rand Corporation and the Subcommittee on Health Insurance of the New York State Council on Health Care Financing, where he aided in the development of New York's new hospital payment system. His primary research interests include evaluations of the impact of public policies on hospital and nursing home behavior. Specific examples include an evaluation of the cost and access implications of alternative hospital payment methodologies in New York's (Medicare) waiver program, the impact of DRG payment on hospital readmission rates, as well as his ongoing research evaluating the RUG–II nursing home payment system in New York. He is a member of the Association for Health Services Research. Dr. Thorpe received his Ph.D. in Public Policy Analysis at the Rand Graduate Institute.

## Contributors

CYNTHIA GREEN is a Senior Research Associate at the Citizens Budget Commission, with primary responsibility for monitoring the finances of New York State. Her research interests are in the areas of state and local finance and social policy. She has authored articles and contributed to edited volumes on New York State's budget, finances, accounting practices, and local assistance. She received a B.A. in Human Development and Family Studies from Cornell University and an M.A. in Urban Affairs and Policy Analysis from the New School for Social Research, and she is a doctoral candidate at New York University's Graduate School of Public Administration.

MARTHA SOLISH is a health policy, health management, and social services consultant. She has worked with hospitals, health maintenance organizations, and ambulatory clinics, with particular emphasis on the problems of public hospitals and the uninsured. She has held management positions with a private health care consulting firm, the Brandeis University Health Policy Center, and the Massachusetts Medicaid program. She is currently president and cofounder of Homeless Women's Housing Initiative, Inc., a not-for-profit developer of permanent and transitional housing for homeless families. Ms. Solish holds M.B.A. and M.P.H. degrees from Columbia University.

JOEL WEISSMAN received his Master of City Planning degree from The Massachusetts Institute of Technology and his Doctorate in Social Welfare, specializing in Health Policy, from the Heller School at Brandeis University. Before his attendance at the Heller School, Dr. Weissman taught health administration courses at the Massachusetts College of Pharmacy. His research experience has covered a variety of topics in health policy and economics, including the costs associated with hospice, the use of controlled drugs by health providers, and studies of health services utilization in public hospital outpatient departments and by uninsured inpatients in the Boston metropolitan area. Dr. Weissman concentrates his research efforts in the area of health services utilization, particularly around those issues associated with access to care and use of health services by disadvantaged populations.